FIRED UP

SUPERCHARGE IMMUNITY, DOUBLE YOUR STRENGTH, LIFT LIBIDO, SHED FAT, AND START FEELING YOUNG AND ALIVE AGAIN

WITH THE UNIQUE SYNERGY OF HIIT, YOGA & STRENGTH TRAINING

INTRODUCTION

The overwhelming desire to feel good, look good and remain youthful has driven the human race to seek methods and strategies for achieving these desires since the beginning of historical records. Some of these methods and strategies have produced flourishing enterprises geared towards enhancing the health of the human race, including 24-hour gyms, yoga studios for all ages, affordable home exercise equipment and supplements that make up for the nutritional deficit in our modern diet.

While many of these enterprises have had a positive impact on human health, the amount of money up for grabs in the worldwide health and wellness industry ($4.2 Trillion as of 2017)[1] combined with the desire for instant gratification has created a breeding ground for charlatans and scammers looking to capitalize and get rich off of ignorant consumers.

Sadly, the ripple effect of an ever-increasing amount of products and services has brought with it a plethora of poor guidance and information, which has contributed to a myopic view of health and set up multiple traps along the road to health and wellness.

Since avoiding this myopic view of health is so important, our first task will be to self reflect and be honest if you've ever fallen into this trap from any products or services you purchased in the past.   Let's take a look at the definition:

Myopic - *lacking in foresight or discernment: narrow in perspective and without concern for broader implications.*

Do you look at labels or think about the long-term effects of things before you purchase and try them? Or do you look at the short-term benefits and jump in without looking at the bigger picture?

While everyone at some point falls into this trap there is **Good News!** In Fired Up our goal is not just short-term gratification (myopic) but long-term wellness and superior human health. This rare but achievable state not only considers the individual elements of mental, physical and emotional health but the combined synergy of the three.

Essentially, by combining these three aspects you'll not only be physically strong and look your best but you'll be more resistant to illness (like Covid-19), better able to cope with stress, and feel more alive with a true zest for life.

In this program, we'll be using a combination of disciplines that will help you develop the capacity to produce superhuman power. Yes, this may sound like a bold promise but I encourage you to suspend your disbelief until after you've completed your first few months of the training. And there's a really good reason for this 90-day mark.

According to studies, 60-90 days is all it takes to create a lifetime habit, [2] which in this case will help you sustain that superhuman power.

So I ask you, wouldn't it be worth going all in 100% on the *Fired Up* program for 90 days to see if it could indeed give you superhuman power for the rest of your life? Really, what's the worst thing that could happen here?

While I can't guarantee you'll follow through and take the recommended action, if you do I can absolutely guarantee you'll feel really good about yourself, you'll accomplish more with superhuman powers that not only make you stronger, faster and more agile but lower less stress and help you sleep like a baby. And if you fear any virus out there I can also guarantee that you'll also have a much better chance at kicking it to the curb by simply following my recommended guidance.

If you need proof let me throw myself into the equation. I got Covid-19, yet it did not seem to effect me anywhere near it affected others. In fact, it seemed like a low grade Flu that kept coming and going for a couple months. I lost my appetite, felt nauseous and couldn't workout as much but it never really crushed me like other Flu viruses of the past. Why?

I don't inherently possess superhuman powers, I've created them with exactly what you're about to learn in this book.

And just what are those superhuman powers you can obtain from the *Fired Up* program? We'll get into the amazing benefits of the program shortly, for now it's important to understand that in order to achieve this synergy of superhuman power and stack the deck in your favor you'll first need to be aware of the pitfalls and traps that lure you away from your goals and prevent you from triumphantly crossing the victory line.   This brings us to the first chapter "The Traps of Triumph."

CHAPTER 1 – THE TRAPS OF TRIUMPH

"The will to win, the desire to succeed, the urge to reach your full potential... these are the keys that will unlock the door to personal excellence." - Confucius

While there are a multitude of circumstances and excuses that could potentially end or delay your quest for personal excellence, none is greater than lack of desire. For this reason, we'll be taking a few extra steps to ensure you reach your ultimate goals.

In regards to those goals and in the interest of keeping you motivated towards achieving them, I'd like you to take a moment right now and imagine you are setting out on a long journey to find your own island full of buried treasure.

When first embarking on this journey you'll need to define two things on the map as follows:

1) Where you are now and…

2) Where you want to go

Without these two pieces of information, you could get lost in the Bermuda Triangle of misguided information or waste a lot of time drifting in a sea with no wind, or perhaps even get attacked by a pack of pirates looking to cash in on your discovery.

Similarly, as you head out to get *"Fired Up"* you'll need to identify where you are now and where you want to go. By identifying these two points you'll see a clear path to victory, set yourself up for success, and stack the deck in your favor.

The first part of this equation – where you are now – is critical as it allows you to identify the obstacles that could make your journey take twice as long or perhaps prevent you from getting there at all.   So here is your first question:

Where am I at in my journey toward optimal health and fitness?

If for instance, you have a lot of inflammation in your body and jump into the recommended exercises, you could actually go backward simply because of the fact that strength training and HIIT add more inflammation. Yes, inflammation serves a good purpose in the tearing down and rebuilding of muscle but inflammation on top of inflammation equals couch crush (AKA your ass stuck on the couch).

We'll talk more about inflammation later, just know for now, we are all unique, with different levels of health and fitness. So as we embark on this journey of building superhuman power you'll need to be really self-honest about where you're at right now in order to get where you want to be in the future.

This brings us to those traps, which either force you to give up shortly after starting or waste valuable time, money and energy. So first, I'm going list several traps below; notice if you've fallen prey to any of them in the past and how this new awareness can lift the fog of delusion and open up a new path to obtaining superhuman powers.

IG (Instant Gratification)

If you're looking at that IG and thinking "Instagram," you're not far off. In fact, Instagram has built an empire on instant gratification, so much so, that we could call it "instant gratification" rather than Instagram. More often than not, we look at a picture or a 10 second video on Instagram and we want what they have and… we want it as quick as possible.

As previously mentioned, with trillions of dollars up for grabs, the health and wellness market has become a breeding ground for scammers who have played (indiscriminately) on our desires for instant gratification by selling us products and services with little regard for our health and safety.

If you're at all short on examples consider one small case from 2014 when the US Federal Trade Commissions cracked down on four multimillion-dollar companies Sensa Products, L'Occitane, HCG Diet Direct and LeanSpa for making "unfounded promises."

In a market of people experiencing epidemic proportions of obesity, the lure of instant weight loss without any effort has become a sort of plague. At its height, the weight loss industry in the US experienced a massive push to sell shady products by making outlandish advertising claims like:

- "Get a gym body without going to the gym" by sprinkling a powder on your food.
- "Significantly slim your thighs and buttocks" using an almond-scented cream.
- "Lose up to one pound a day with just two drops under the tongue."

Such claims were deceptive, according to the Federal Trade Commission, who ordered the four companies to collectively pay $34 million in refunds to consumers.

Of course, this is just one example of thousands of scams and rip-offs that have left consumers wondering who to trust.

Solution to Instant Gratification

If there is no work involved in creating something amazing I can pretty much guarantee it's a scam. As such, you'll need to remember this one:

If it sounds too good to be true it probably is!

And

No effort = No reward!

The Guru Trap

While there are clearly unscrupulous people in the health and wellness world making millions of dollars selling stuff that isn't really helping you, there are legitimate experts who have good intentions but fall into another trap I like to call "The Guru Trap."

This happens when a really smart expert in a particular field finds a method or substance that provides a great benefit to both themselves and to their clients and as a result gains notoriety and fame.

While notoriety and fame are not inherently bad, if you start believing everything someone says simply because they are famous or educated with a doctoral degree there is a great risk for falling for the Guru Trap and being deceived.

Most of us have heard of cult gurus like L Ron Hubbard, Charles Manson and Bhagwan Shree Rajneesh but gurus from the health industry can have cult like status as well.

Bikram Choudhury was famous for popularizing hot yoga in America. Yet, despite the amazing benefits of the practice, people began worshipping him as a godhead figure and allowed themselves to be taken advantage of. He was eventually tried and convicted of sexual misconduct, raping and sexually assaulting several of his students and has since fled the country where he remains a fugitive.

Or take Dr. Atkins for instance. Atkins was famous for the Atkins diet, which allowed people to eat mostly protein and fat while restricting carbohydrates.

Unfortunately, the diet is marketed with questionable claims that carbohydrate restriction is critical to weight loss.[3] While I and other experts agree with this to a certain extent, studies also show that too much protein can lead to weight gain.[4]

In summary, there is no good evidence of the diet's effectiveness in achieving long-term weight loss[5] and it may in fact, increase the risk of heart disease.[6]

Nevertheless, since the Guru (Dr. Atkins) was a famous doctor, and people got short-term weight loss benefits, people jumped on the bandwagon despite the risks.

But even more disturbing is the fact that people still follow the diet today despite their guru himself being grossly overweight and purportedly dying of a heart attack.

What's even more interesting is the fact that Dr. Atkins had a long history of heart attacks and congestive heart failure and when he died his wife cremated his body before an autopsy could be completed.

Question: Would you jump off a 3,000-foot cliff just because a famous doctor told you it would be ok? Of course, you wouldn't. I'd imagine you'd probably do a little research to see if the claims the guru made were legitimate and make an educated decision.

So why would you follow the advice of a doctor just because he paid for a $50,000 education.

Solution To The Guru Trap

When starting a new diet or exercise program, it's absolutely critical to make sure the program is backed not only by long-term scientific studies (which may not be available) but other experts who are trustworthy.

Fortunately, Fired Up is backed by multiple experts and long-term studies, which prove its undeniable power.

The One Way Trap

Similar to the Guru Trap, the One Way Trap is usually promoted by a small group or individual as a superior discipline to everyone else's.

When this happens the promoter of the "one way" typically possesses a large capacity in one area but very limited in other areas. As a result of this myopic mindset the Guru typically shuts down any possibility that there may be a better way than their own.

This is the "my way or the highway" approach; the guy or gal who tells you to ditch everything you're doing because they've found the Holy Grail of health.

For example, I recently read a strength-training book by an MD and a well-known gym trainer that claimed: "you don't need yoga." Unfortunately, they failed to back up this statement with any scientific studies or acknowledge the fact that yoga is one of the oldest, most popular and most beneficial forms of exercise known to mankind (predating weightlifting by several thousand years).

It's understandable when someone gets benefit from something that they would want to shout from the rooftops and share their benefits. Unfortunately, overzealous zealots rarely find the Holy Grail of health or anything of lasting value for that matter.

When we take a look at some of the more recent developments in the fitness world we find a lot of buzz around HIIT (AKA high intensity interval training) and for good reason. When performed properly it has the ability to deliver the same benefits of a 90 – 120 minute workout (low intensity jogging, walking or cycling) in 5% of the time. And while this awesome time saving feature may sound like the best thing since gluten free bread, what most people don't understand is that no matter how great your exercise routine is or how little you need to do it, sitting for excessively long periods of time could kill you.

Yes, that's right, the longer you sit, the higher you are at risk of an early death, regardless of how much you exercise. And to assure you I'm not just a hypocrite hammering gurus while making more unfounded claims, I'd like to direct your attention to a landmark study of 7,985 adults published in Annals of Internal Medicine. In this study, researchers found a direct relationship between time spent sitting and your risk of early mortality of any cause regardless of exercise.[7]

In other words, even if you manage to find an awesome exercise program like HIIT, which takes only 15 minutes a day three days a week to get amazing benefits, if you're sitting for the rest of the time, chances are you won't be feeling so awesome.

Sadly, these myopic views of health aren't just found in weight lifting or high intensity interval training but can be found just about everywhere you turn. This includes disciplines on the opposite end of the spectrum like yoga or tai chi, where gurus can be found claiming their superiority over all other disciplines.

So while each guru from each discipline may display some amazing results, testimonials, and scientific data to back up their claims (a lot of which is legitimate) it's important to look at the bigger picture and not get hung up on one myopic way.

Solution to the One Way Trap

Whatever you've heard in the past, whatever your beliefs are in the present, I want to encourage you right now to suspend them for a moment and open up your mind to a new world of unlimited possibilities.

If there is one major lesson I've learned which is effective 100% of the time it's this:

There is no single person or guru who has all the answers!

Remember, we are all human and as such we have flaws (myself included). Once you truly understand that nobody is perfect, you can begin to expand, open to new solutions and achieve true greatness. Most importantly, right now it's time to embrace a new more powerful philosophy:

Learning and growing is the key to success!

This isn't just fluffy cheerleader pep talk either. If you read my book "Get High On Confidence" you may remember a study conducted by Dr. Carol Dweck, which I'll share here.

In the first study, 373 7th graders demonstrated that students who believed intelligence was malleable (AKA Growth Mindset) showed an improvement in grades over the two years of junior high school, while those with a belief that intelligence is fixed (AKA Fixed Mindset) showed a decline in grades over the same period.[8]

In the second study, an intervention was created in order to teach the growth mindset, which promoted positive change in classroom motivation compared with a control group. Simultaneously, students in the control group displayed a continuing downward trajectory in grades, while this decline was reversed for students in the experimental group.

In conclusion, researchers noted: "The key message was that learning changes the brain by forming new connections and that students are in charge of this process."

So what does this mean for you?

These and other similar studies show that people with a "Fixed Mindset" believe that making a leap forward to acquire a skill or level of intelligence they don't currently have is difficult to impossible. When they see an obstacle, instead of moving towards it, they withdraw and conclude that they are not capable. And while many will view this as a lack of motivation or laziness, more often than not, it's usually just a case of a fixed mindset.

In contrast, people who have a "Growth Mindset" believe that the way to leap forward and succeed is to learn and grow. When they see an obstacle, they move towards it and conclude that if they learn and grow they can become capable and succeed.

In reality, the most advanced humans are advanced because they've learned multiple disciplines from multiple perspectives and multiple teachers. This has been my philosophy for the last 20 years, over which I've accumulated and continue to accumulate skills, abilities and strategies from the masters of multiple disciplines and will share with you throughout this training. Ultimately, this means you get the benefits without having to spend 20 years of your life and

$100,000 figuring out the answers to building superhuman power.

So I urge you to stay open to learning and growing. Your mental and physical abilities are certainly not set and can expand tremendously with a broader perspective and time tested wisdom to gain new results.

The Comfort Zone

Ahh yes, the good old comfort zone. Ever wake up and find yourself saying something like, I don't feel motivated to workout so I'm just going to eat instead? Or maybe you've been working all day and you find yourself thinking, I've been working all day, I deserve to relax, sit on the couch and eat treats, savory dishes, and maybe a glass of beer or wine.

While there will be times for relaxing and relaxing is important, more often than not, falling prey to the comfort zone is really just a distraction from doing the things that will make you really feel good – without negative side effects.

Solution to the Comfort Zone

Fortunately, habits can be changed and to solve this life-crushing trap, we'll be using some ninja tools to change the root of the problem. So instead of drinking three cups of coffee or throwing your TV out the window to get motivated, we'll be addressing the root of the problem - your underlying beliefs.

And by the time you finish this program, instead of falling prey to couch crush, you'll be much more inclined to take action and move your body because you'll get an unmatched high from getting *"Fired Up"* that simply can't be replaced by food, drugs or TV.

Overkill

I'd imagine you're anxious to dive in and start building superhuman power but before we do I strongly encourage you to hold off for one more moment in order to save yourself from our final trap – Overkill.

A lot of my clients are eager to jump in headfirst and get started. While I admire this enthusiasm if you're not ready for a certain level of exercise you could injure yourself and just end up back on the sidelines as a prisoner to couch crush.

Question: Have you ever tried something new and had a negative experience?

I can't tell you how many hundreds of people have complained of fitness programs that made them never want to return. I'm going to list a few examples below; as you read them, notice if any relate to a situation you've experienced in the past.

- My first yoga class was brutal because the teacher didn't know what they were doing and I threw my back out.

- I went to my first HIIT class, which was 60 minutes long and I felt like throwing up.

- I did a routine strength training exercise and was sore for seven days.

Can you find the common thread between these examples? If you guessed overkill, you're right. But before you dismiss this as unimportant and miss out on some of the greatest treasures of life, make sure you familiarize yourself with the three primary factors that create it.

The 3 Factors of Overkill

1) Lack of Proper Instruction - First, without proper instruction to guide you gradually towards optimal health, you may injure yourself and give up. So I want to take this moment to advise that you take into consideration your current health and fitness level.

If you are new to a particular discipline you'll need to really listen to instructions and shoot for gradual improvement rather than overnight superhuman strength.

2) The Lesser Ego - Second, regardless of who you learn from, if starting at the bottom isn't something you're willing to do because it makes you look bad in front of others, you're in for a very long and painful road ahead.

As a yoga instructor for over 14 years, I've watched countless inexperienced men and women attempt something way out of their ability level and not only make a fool of themselves but injure themselves at the same time.   So I encourage you to let go of your smaller ego that needs to be at the top immediately and embrace your greater self by shooting for gradual progression towards superhuman strength.

3) Confusing Fitness with Health - Both modern and ancient societies have glorified both the beauty and power of muscle and endurance since the times of ancient Greece when perfectly chiseled statues graced the city streets of Athens around the year 700 B.C. While these statues were created to commemorate great athletes who accomplished great feats and soldiers who gave their lives in the service of others, ultimately this laid the foundation for the ideal body regardless of whether or not it created optimal health.

Fast forward roughly 2,500 years into the 18th Century and we find weightlifting as an official competition and entertainment spectacle where strongmen who would risk their lives by picking up cars or dragging a train to please a crowd.

Naturally, weightlifting continued to progress and through much evolution became an official event in the Olympics where an athlete's sole goal is to lift as much weight as possible one time. Unfortunately, this goal has little to do with creating optimal health.

And while weightlifting for sport may have had a measurable winner – he who lifts the most wins – with the advent of bodybuilding came an entire sport, which used neither strength, endurance, or health as any of its primary objectives. Instead, it's primary goal lies in the quest for perfect symmetry and muscular monstrosity most famously demonstrated by one of its greatest statues - Arnold Schwarzenegger.

Perhaps even more vexing is the endurance world. If we simply retrace the origins of the long distance race called "Marathon" we find the story of a Greek messenger named Pheidippides who ran from a city called Marathon to Athens (26.2 miles) to deliver news of a military victory against the Persians at the Battle of Marathon. Now can you guess what happened to him after he delivered his message?

He died on the spot. It should be noted, however, that Pheidippides did run an addition 150 miles (estimated) over two days prior to his run to Marathon.

Despite this account and dozens of studies, which prove running for long distances to be harmful to your long-term health, millions of people make running a Marathon as one of their primary goals in life.

Even worse, ultra marathon runners, who complete similar feats as Pheidippides did, are seen as godlike. That is of course until they get ill or die from over exhaustion.

When we look at the most notable people in the fitness world like world class athletes and bodybuilders, we are conditioned by society to believe that being fit somehow equates to being healthy and the more fit you are the more healthy you will become. Unfortunately, being more fit only helps you become healthier to a certain degree.

If you struggle with this concept at all think about it this way. Your heart only has so many beats per life. Nobody knows exactly how many you have and we are all unique, but no one can dispute this fact. This doesn't just apply to your heartbeats but your muscles, bones, brain cells, cartilage and everything else that holds you together. If you use all your available resources over a short period of time (overkill), sorry but you just aren't going to live that long, nor will you have optimal health.

Solution To Overkill

The solution to overkill is again to follow the training manual and honor yourself whatever level you're at. Fortunately, the *Fired Up* manual and video program will guide you step-by-step in choosing the best program for your current ability level and get you to the "where you want to go" part of that road map.

The Destination – Your Goal

This brings us to the "where you want to go" part of the treasure map, which is the goal of this training. But before we identify that place let's first get clear about **what this training is not**.

- The goal of this training is not to make you look like a bodybuilder who can neither touch their toes nor maneuver around obstacles because they have limited their range of motion from a disproportionate amount of muscle.

- The goal of this training is not to make you so fit you can run 100 miles or do 60 minutes of high intensity interval training while creating more injuries and reducing your life span.

- The goal of this training is not to make you shrivel up into a bendy pretzel so you can put your foot behind your head or do a handstand.

- Most importantly, the goal is this training is not to become fit at the expense of optimal health.

With that out of the way let's now get clear on **what this training is.** Our overall goal in *Fired Up* is to develop optimal health, which does the following:

- Makes you **feel alive with youthful energy**.

- Makes you **strong and powerful, physically and mentally**.

- Creates flexible muscles across your entire body, which makes you **more mobile, nimble, agile and less vulnerable to injuries.**

- **Optimizes your mental capacity** so you can withstand the onslaught of stress presented by your environment, which in turn **increases your lifespan**.

- Allows you to **shed unnecessary body fat and feel confident about yourself** because you're at your ideal body weight. Ideal body weight, in turn, boosts your immune system and allows you to crush illnesses like the coronavirus.

- **Gives you a constant source of pure energy** that makes you **maximally productive** so you can get way more done in much less time.

Why Listen To Me?

If you're not familiar with my books or trainings you may be asking yourself, "Why should I listen to you?"

Personally, I've spent most of my life studying and practicing different athletic disciplines, which also brought with them a plethora of injuries, healing modalities, therapists, coaches and accompanying lessons.

My first dream was to play in the NFL, but that dream was crushed. Literally, in my second year as a wide receiver at San Diego State University, I jumped up to catch a pass and was blindsided by a 260-pound Samoan linebacker who crushed my sternal clavicular joint with his helmet and ended my football career.

Originally having grown up in the Colorado Rockies, my next dream was to be a professional mogul skier, but that dream was torn apart. Literally, in my third year of college, I skipped school to go on a ski trip and at the end of the day over rotated on a 360 aerial maneuver. When my body landed it continued to rotate but the ski, which was attached to my leg, did not, which tore my MCL, ACL and meniscus in my left knee.

But sports was my passion and even though I would never fully recover from that knee injury, I somehow convinced myself I could snowboard my way to the podium since this sport didn't have the lateral risks associated with my injury. As you can imagine from the way this story is going, it didn't end well.

After launching myself off a ramp I landed on my shoulder, which sent me back to the operating table to sew up a torn rotator cuff

with a few metal pins to add to my collection
of battle scars.

Fortunately, or unfortunately (depending
on your belief system), I had one last run in
with the ER (emergency room) when I
attempted to break the record for time to run
up and down Cowls Mountain in San Diego.

Can you guess what happened?

Yep… this also ended in major trauma!

Turns out the trail was lined with slippery
gravel and about half way down I found
myself heading face first into the ground
without any feet underneath me. My natural
instinct was to put my arm out and brace for
impact but since I had been traveling at
breakneck speed (pun intended), when my
arm hit the ground the force of gravity broke
the head of my humorous clean of my arm.

Basically, my arm was dangling from my
shoulder, being held together by little more
than ligaments, tendons and skin.

Fortunately, (again, depending on your
belief system) all trauma holds within it an
opportunity for learning, growth, development
and change. For me, there were two giant
life lessons from these traumas that
catapulted me forward to my true calling in
life.

First and foremost, my path was not to be
a professional athlete. All signs pointed in
the direction of creation and contribution,
which led me to music and personal
development, my passion and mission,
respectively.

Second, all this trauma forced me to learn
about healing, rebuilding and strengthening

without succumbing to my new handicaps – a permanently jacked up knee, clavicle joint and shoulder. By this time I had seen more physical therapists, trainers and doctors than one could realistically expect to see in several lifetimes.

Over the last 25 years these experts and therapists along with my own investigation and training exposed me to the most advanced tools and techniques for building health and fitness in ways I never imagined.

What I discovered was three powerful disciplines that when combined created a synergistic effect unrivaled by anything I'd ever experienced before. This, of course, was the combination of Yoga, HIIT and Strength Training.

By combining these three disciplines along with a specific diet called "***The Power Diet***," my health improved from lackluster in my 20's and 30's to robust and vibrant in my 40's and beyond.

Now I don't get sick or injured as often, I feel energized throughout the day and I'm productive all the way until bedtime. My mind is clear and answers come to me quickly. My testosterone levels are as high as they were in my 30's and my libido is noticeably more potent since I implemented these programs.

So get excited, because if you simply follow the recommended action in this program you too will be able to build unlimited power and feel like a superhuman.

CHAPTER 2 – THE SYNERGY OF 3

Synergy – *"The interaction or cooperation of two or more organizations, substances, or other agents to produce a combined effect greater than the sum of their separate effects."*

Clearly a myopic view of exercise and fitness, or life in general, rarely solves the root of the problem and creates optimal health.   So instead of limiting ourselves to one discipline or one belief, in *Fired Up,* we'll be branching out, expanding, and increasing our health, fitness, confidence, power and longevity by combining three of the most powerful disciplines available - HIIT, Yoga and Strength Training.

Why These Three?

There are literally hundreds of different exercise disciplines to choose from so why would the combination of HIIT, Yoga, and Strength Training create the ultimate formula for superhuman power?

The Triad of Optimal Health

Remember, our goal is not just fitness, it's optimal health. If you've read my book "Get High On Confidence," you may remember "The Triad of Unbreakable Confidence," which includes your physical, mental and spiritual confidence.

Similarly, you can't have optimal health without these three key components of physical, mental and spiritual health, which together create what I call: "The Triad of Superhuman Strength."

Now if for any reason the word spiritual makes you feel uneasy, don't worry, we're not going get all woo-woo here and talk about religion. What we are going to do though is acknowledge and harness the unseen power of your mind.

For example, while HIIT and Strength Training do not offer much if any spiritual or mental power, yoga does. In fact, one of the definitions of yoga is "union between mind and body," the power of which cannot be underestimated. If you're not already hip to this, it's been well documented that the stress, which comes from your mind, can create illness in your body.[9]

If, for example, you had a rough day at the office and/or your relationship is in turmoil you may find that the stress in your mind then translates into illness in your body which may manifest as an unexplained cough or sudden onset of flu like symptoms.

Another quite common example of this union of mind and body is the reason why most people give up on training programs. More often than not, they do so simply because their mind and its belief systems do not support the continued discipline it takes to follow through and create a long-term habit. This has been demonstrated scientifically on multiple occasions.

If you're at all skeptical, consider the famous TV show "The Biggest Loser." Results reported from Reuters Health stated that six years after dramatic weight loss on the TV show most contestants had regained the pounds. In addition, the study showed contestants' metabolisms had slowed and they were burning fewer calories every day than they did before their stint on the show.

Six years later, when the six men and eight women went to the National Institutes of Health for follow-up measurements, their weight, on average, was back up to 290 pounds. Only one participant had not regained any weight.[10]

Essentially, if you do not address your mind you will always be limited to how much you can develop your body.

Fortunately, as mentioned earlier, we'll be digging out the toxic roots of this trap and getting rid of this problem with some highly effective strategies.

They Complement Each Other

What is most miraculous about these three disciplines is how elegantly they complement and enhance one another. Let's explore the synergistic effects in detail so you clearly understand how committing to a long-term practice can create superhuman power for you.

Yoga Makes Everything Easier, Safer And More Effective!

If for instance, you love going to the gym and strength training, you may find yourself having a hard time keeping your lower back in a neutral (safe) position when descending into a squat. If this is the case, there's a good chance your hamstrings are too tight, which is where yoga comes in big since it can help release this tension and make you more flexible, agile and mobile; not to mention save you from a painful injury.

Or let's say you love HIIT but you find your right shoulder is in pain. There is a good chance you may have tight fascia. As a connective tissue, which covers all of your muscles, fascia is commonly overlooked because you cannot see it, nor does it make you look superhuman. Unfortunately, without addressing this critical part of your anatomy you could get injured or remain in pain for a very long time.

More often than not, when you do a balanced yoga routine like the ones offered in *Fired Up* you'll be stretching and releasing tension in your muscles and the fascia that wrap your feet, legs, back, shoulders and arms. As a result, you may find a longstanding pain that just wouldn't seem to leave is no longer causing you pain.

This is the power of yoga. It addresses a multitude of health markers that neither HIIT nor strength training can.

But perhaps yoga's most far-reaching benefit is its ability to reduce stress by stimulating your parasympathetic nervous system (PNS) and deactivating your sympathetic nervous system (SNS).   This is highly significant, since modern societal stressors like jobs, family, and finances are constantly triggering your SNS and according to studies, is considered one of the biggest contributors to illness and disease. In fact, studies show that as many as 80% of all doctors' visits for maladies such as colds, flu viruses, migraine headaches and IBS (irritable bowel syndrome) are stress related.[11] [12] [13] [14]

Fortunately, yoga, when properly instructed, turns on your SNS and slows down your heart rate, lowers your blood pressure, and reduces cortisol.   The result of these functions can be found in the peaceful bliss and clear headed thinking that comes right after practicing. This, in turn, eliminates negative mental chatter that drives people to mindlessly overreact, over consume, over spend and end up on the couch defeated with couch crush.

In contrast, HIIT and Strength training, simply don't address these optimal health factors, which makes yoga an invaluable team member of The Triad of Superhuman Strength.

Strength Training Protects Joints And Adds Stability

Of course, strength training has its own unique benefits, which can boost your Yoga or HIIT practice to a whole new level.

If for instance, you love yoga but you struggle with chaturanga or can't do an arm balance, strength training can give you both the stability and strength to safely move through these more challenging postures without risking injury.

HIIT Builds Testosterone And HGH

If you practice yoga but you just can't seem to boost your HGH or Testosterone to optimal levels, both HIIT and Strength Training, when done according to the *Fired Up* protocol, have been proven to maximize levels of these critical superhuman hormones.

Synergy Of 3 Provides Anaerobic & Aerobic Benefits

One of the greatest benefits of combining these three disciplines lies in the fact that they address the two main categories of exercise - aerobic and anaerobic. Let's explore both aerobic and anaerobic systems briefly so you have a better understanding of why this is so important.

Aerobic is defined as:

"Involving or improving oxygen consumption by the body"

In other words, aerobic exercise enhances respiratory and circulatory efficiency by improving oxygen consumption. Aerobic movements require oxygen to generate force and activate slow-twitch muscles for activity over sustained periods of time (typically several minutes). Most experts believe constant movement of 8 minutes or more qualifies as aerobic exercise.

Some good examples of aerobic exercise would include methods that do not alternate pace much like jogging, swimming, cycling, and aerobic gym classes. Surprisingly, according to several studies, if done with enough intensity, yoga can also be considered aerobic.[15] [16]

In contrast, anaerobic means:

"Without oxygen (does not require oxygen to generate force)"

Anaerobic movements activate fast-twitch muscles for short bursts of intense activity for short durations of time (from a few seconds to a minute). Some good examples of anaerobic exercises include anything that pushes your heart rate close to its maximum for a few seconds to a minute. This could be anything from high intensity weight lifting, calisthenics, swimming, cycling or sprinting, depending on whether or not you create intervals and vary the pace.   And again, depending on the program, yoga can once again be considered anaerobic.

Clearly, there are many ways to do both Aerobic and Anaerobic exercise. The question is: how can we get the benefits of both without having to over tax our bodies or switch from one discipline to the next in the same workout?

For many years people believed a significant increase in fitness could only be achieved through endurance training until a study in 2008 proved this false.[17] Essentially, researchers demonstrated scientifically that a HIIT program consisting of four to six 30-second maximal cycling sprints, followed by 4.5 minute recovery bouts, three days per week provided similar increases in levels of oxidative enzymes as those who performed 40 – 60 minutes of steady cycling at 65% VO2max five days per week.

In summary, the study proved that 6 - 9 minutes of HIIT per week created the same benefits of aerobic exercise for 200 - 300 minutes per week. This was a major discovery and turned the fitness world on its head.

Since this and other studies clearly demonstrate the possibility for activation of aerobic and anaerobic systems in one exercise we'll be taking advantage of this by incorporating several different variations of Strength Training, Yoga and HIIT.

And while diet and sleep are also major factors for optimal health (which we'll talk about later), these three disciplines form an unmatched synergy, which creates The Triad of Superhuman Strength.

My Promise To You

I guarantee that no matter what you look like right now, no matter where you come from or what your history is, if you can hunker down, read each word and take the action recommended in the *Fired Up* program, you will transform your mind and body to feel superhuman. This will then translate into a feeling of being powerful, strong, energetic, and confident, which will radiate to the world around you and attract loads of love and respect.

CHAPTER 3 – FIX THE ROOT

"The battles that count aren't the ones for gold medals. The struggles within yourself… the invisible, inevitable battles inside all of us… that's where it's at."   – Jesse Owens

While this next chapter may not directly affect the transformation of your biceps, triceps or abs, it will indirectly affect the outcome of every muscle in your body. Essentially, this is all about the master and captain who are guiding your ship and will determine whether or not you find your treasure of superhuman power.

Now can you guess who the master and captain are?

These powerful individuals guide your every move, determine your results (or lack thereof) and represent your beliefs that reside in your mind. This is the most crucial power source of all, which could either lead you into a pack of pirates or to your island full of treasure, so stay focused here.

Remember how I mentioned earlier in "The Comfort Zone" how most people who try a new diet or exercise program fail? Well, this is your golden opportunity to beat the odds and end up on that 10% side of the scale instead of the 90% who die with loads of regrets.

I like to think of the reason why most people fail at instituting a new regimen into their life is similar to the challenge of killing a weed. If you simply hack off the branches and everything above the ground, the roots will remain intact and eventually grow back. Yo-yo diets are a perfect example of this phenomenon.

We mentioned the show the Biggest Loser but for every loser on that show, we can guesstimate that at least 100,000 other people also lost the battle of the bulge.

My client Greg really wanted to lose weight, boost his testosterone and find a wife, but each time he tried a new diet and exercise program he lost some weight but eventually, a few months or a few years later, he gained it all back.   But why does this happen so frequently?

As martial arts master Bruce Lee once famously declared:

"As you think so shall you be"

If you've been through my groundbreaking training <u>The Winner's Mindset</u> you'll have learned that the only way to solve any problem is to address the root, which represents your belief about something. This has now been scientifically proven and documented by therapists like the founder of Cognitive Behavioral Therapy Dr. Aaron T Beck and confirmed over thousands of years by Sages like Buddha, Jesus and Socrates.

For example, if you believe Strength Training is boring and painful you probably won't ever go to the gym. Or if you believe yoga is really just for women and you're not limber enough to do it you probably won't commit long enough to make it a lifetime habit. Or if you believe that HIIT is too exhausting and only for top athletes you most likely will never start.

But if you believed that Strength Training, Yoga and HIIT are a celebration of what your body can do and makes you feel superhuman, you'll look forward to working out and you'll get addicted to it (in a good way).

To better understand this I've created a model by which all results are created called the Circle of Results Model and here is how it works.

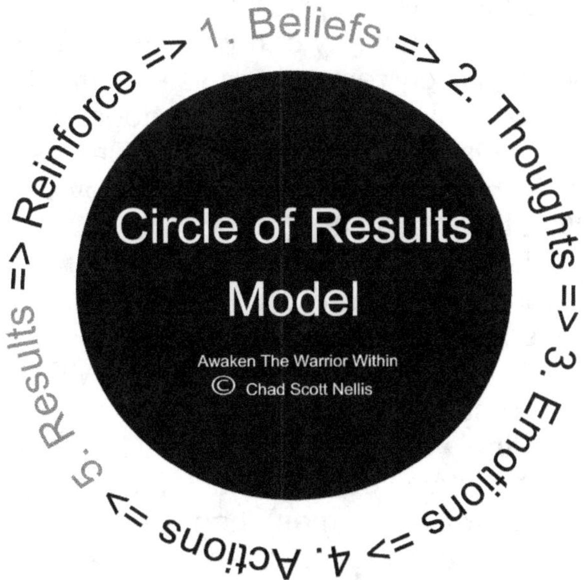

As you can see from the Circle of Results Model diagram:

Beliefs   =>   Thoughts
Thoughts =>   Emotions
Emotions =>   Actions
Actions   =>   Results
Results   =>   Reinforce Beliefs

Think about that circle of results for a second. Each time you think, "it's too painful," it actually creates an emotion of fear, which leads to inaction. As a consequence of inaction, your result leaves you stuck with the same weak and powerless body, which then reinforces your disempowered belief and gets hard-wired into your brain – it's too painful! And the more you do this, the more difficult it is to undo or rewire this belief.

If you've read any of my previous books you most likely remember this statement: "Neurons that fire together wire together," which was also made famous by Dr. Joe Dispenza, a neuroscientist in the movie "What the Bleep Do We Know."

This is how your brain works. Your neurons in your brain are the wires that connect associated memories with experiences you've had in the past, which then create your beliefs. So if you believe every time you go work out you'll just feel pain (because you did, in fact, feel pain or soreness several times) then your brain will fire off the association wires of "working out" equals "pain" and strengthen its bond. This is the main reason why people fail to stick to diets and exercise programs.

Fortunately, by changing your beliefs we can break the negative chain reaction and create an entirely different result – superhuman strength!

If you have any doubts about the ability to grow new brain cells and rewire your brain, consider the following scientific study.

In 1998, the journal *Nature Medicine* published a report indicating that neurogenesis, the growth of new brain cells, does indeed occur in humans.[18] This monumental discovery overturned generations of conventional wisdom in neuroscience.

Basically, your brain is not limited to the neurons from your childhood and their associated beliefs and by changing your beliefs you can rewire your brain to create superhuman strength.

Now can you guess what else rewires your brain? Hint: It's all about the Triad of Superhuman Strength. Let me explain.

Essentially, neurogenesis is controlled by your DNA (specific gene codes for the production of a protein called BDNF or brain-derived neurotrophic factor (BDNF), which plays a key role in creating new neurons. Interestingly enough, studies reveal decreased BDNF in Alzheimer's patients, as well as in a variety of neurological conditions including epilepsy, depression, schizophrenia and obsessive-compulsive disorder.

Fortunately, many of the factors that influence our DNA to produce BDNF are under our direct control and the gene that turns on BDNF is activated by physical exercise, caloric restriction, curcumin and the omega-3 fat DHA, all of which are included in the *Fired Up* and *The Power Diet programs*.

In fact, laboratory rats that exercise have been shown to produce far more BDNF in their brains compared to sedentary animals. And there is a direct relationship between elevation of BDNF levels in these animals and their ability to learn, as one might expect.

With this understanding of the relationship between BDNF and exercise, researchers also found that elderly individuals engaged in regular physical exercise for a 24-week period had an improvement of an astounding 1,800 percent on measures of memory, language ability, attention and other important cognitive functions compared to an age-matched group not involved in the exercise program.[19]

The mechanism by which exercise enhances brain performance is described in these and other studies as directly related to increased production of BDNF, which brings us back to the goal of this training.

By simply engaging in regular physical exercise using the synergy of yoga, HIIT and strength training, you'll not only become strong, powerful and confident, but your mind will become quick, agile and efficient, which in turn (remember the Circle of Results?) allows you to manifest your most sought after desires.

Pattern Interrupt

With this encouraging outlook and motivation behind us, let's go ahead and handle any potentially self-sabotaging beliefs that stand in the way of you and your superhuman powers.

The first thing to understand about beliefs is that habitually thinking the same negative thing over and over is a negative pattern; sort of like a groove in a broken record that plays over and over.

In order to break any physical neural connections you have associated with negative patterns you'll need to interrupt this pattern by creating a more empowering belief. With this in mind, let's take a look at a Circle of Results model for an average person's health. As you read, make sure you take note if any of this relates to your own personal circumstances and any past failures.

B – I believe that my health isn't that important because I'm not an athlete or anything special. I believe health food tastes horrible and it's expensive. I believe exercising is painful. I don't believe I have time to exercise.

T – I think, I'm going to die anyway, what's the point of putting all this effort into my body. I'm not worth the investment. I'll just stop at McDonalds and grab a quick bite so I can save money and not have to cook anything.

E – I feel sluggish, slow, sick and depressed.

A – I overeat a lot by indulging in fast food, potato chips, snacks and desserts, which probably aren't the best for my health. I just go back and eat the same thing because it's easy and cheap.

R – I'm overweight and have a hard time sleeping and getting out of bed. I don't have the energy to exercise so I usually just watch a lot of television when I get home at night. My dreams keep slipping further and further away because I don't have the energy to take action. I hang out with other people who have low standards and we complain together.

Obviously, this isn't the result we're looking for or anything even close to *"Fired Up,"* so in order to get a different result we'll be using a timeless strategy called modeling taken from my training The Winner's Mindset. By modeling the beliefs of people who have the results we want we can create a newly empowered belief and change our results. Pay attention to the following mindsets and notice, which resonate most with you.

"Exercise is a celebration of what you're body can do not punishment for what you ate." – Author unknown

"Health is your greatest wealth" – Author unknown

*"Let food be
thy medicine and medicine be thy food."* - **Hippocrates**

"Eating well and exercising shows you love and respect yourself while eating unhealthy and remaining sedentary shows you just don't like yourself that much." – Author unknown

"Take care of your body, it's the only place you have to live." - Personal development pioneer Jim Rohn

"To keep the body in good health is a duty... otherwise we shall not be able to keep our mind strong and clear." - The historical Buddha Shakyamuni

German writer and statesman Johann Wolfgang von Goethe was one of the rare giants of world literature. He composed literary works and established artistic principles that had a profound influence on his contemporaries throughout Europe including Napoleon Bonaparte, which are studied today. Goethe proclaimed:

"Take care of your body with steadfast fidelity. The soul must see through these eyes alone, and if they are dim, the whole world is clouded."

Question: Did you notice the common thread of most of these master mindsets?

The common thread is that they all relate back to the unbreakable law of the oneness of mind and body!

In other words, your body is directly connected to your mind (and vise versa) and by engaging regularly in the *Fired Up* program you'll be much more likely to avoid some of those life crushing diseases like Alzheimer's, cancer, atherosclerosis, dementia and the Coronavirus.

Obviously, this is crucial for not only optimal health but human survival, so make absolutely sure you keep this front and center of your mind when it comes time to write down your new beliefs.

Perhaps even more important than avoiding disease is that by seeing the world clearly, as Goethe proclaimed, you can better serve others, create more value and contribute more to the world.

By using the pain of illness and the pleasure of creating superhuman power and contributing more to the world as motivating factors, you'll avoid becoming the biggest loser and instead become the biggest winner - free of regrets!

Later on, we'll be using these leveraging factors to create a new Circle of Results Model for your beliefs, so keep these in mind as possibilities for your newly enhanced superhuman belief system.

CHAPTER 4 –STRENGTH TRAINING

"Strength does not come from winning. Your struggles develop your strengths." – Arnold Schwarzenegger

Strength is a loaded word, which holds within it the potential for increased power on many fronts. Fortunately, by building physical strength we undergo a struggle, which in turn develops our mental strength. At the most basic level, this process begins with "Strength Training," a type of physical exercise specializing in the use of resistance to induce muscular contraction, which then breaks down muscle fibers and rebuilds them through a process known as sarcoplasmic hypertrophy.

With rest and the assistance of protein synthesis (consuming food with protein), studies show strength training creates muscle growth in as little as 2-4 hours of completing a workout.[20] The end result of this process is more strength, anaerobic endurance, and increased size of skeletal muscles.

But strength training isn't just limited to lifting weights in the gym and can be achieved through resistance bands or body weight. So if the gym isn't your thing, don't sweat it because I'm also going to show you how to strength train at home with little to no equipment.

The Awesomeness

Strength training has been studied extensively and its benefits are one of the most well documented of all exercise methods. But if you put all those benefits aside and focus on daily living, you may just find life is easier. And… it feels really empowering when you're stronger.

The need for strength plays out daily in scenarios like carrying groceries, moving the furniture, carrying luggage or picking up your woman (or man) and throwing them on the bed.

Of course, this is just the tip of the iceberg as strength training lifts the awesomeness factor even further with some incredible benefits. As you read the benefits below don't just read them. Instead, imagine them as part of your life and what that would feel like. Again, how you read relates directly to the mental mastery necessary in keeping you committed for life, so don't skip out here.

Gives You Motivation To Follow Your Passions

By delivering a cascade of feel good chemicals like testosterone and serotonin, strength training gives you more motivation and confidence to go after your dreams. This is really significant, since pursuing your dreams could be the most important pursuit of your life.

If you're at all doubtful of this statement, consider the study and documentation from palliative care nurse Bronnie Ware who has cared for thousands of people at the end of their lives. In her book "The Top Regrets of the Dying" she listed the #1 regret at the end of life as doing what others expected instead of doing what you love most.

Fortunately, strength training gives you the motivation to go after your dreams so you don't fall into the graveyard of broken dreams.

Boosts Testosterone

When maximum muscle volume is activated, as taught in the *Fired Up* program, strength training builds testosterone more than any other exercise. Several studies back this up including one published in European Journal of Applied Physiology and Occupational Physiology, which reported a 21.6% in crease in T levels from one 30-minute weightlifting session for men and 16.7% for women.[21]

Another study found that significant increases in the Big T in both young and older men after three sets of lifting weights with slightly larger gains in human growth hormone by the younger men.[22]

Delivering an even bigger bonus (pun intended), studies also show that more testosterone increases libido, erections, energy and cardiovascular health.[23]

Is Testosterone Good For Women?

Confusingly, many people consider testosterone as a hormone exclusive to males yet in reality it's actually crucial for both men and women's health.

For example, studies show that low libido in both men and women is frequently linked to low testosterone.[24] [25] In fact, lack of Testosterone and its associated low libido in women is so prevalent (estimated up to 20 % of all women) there's even a name for it – Hypoactive Sexual Desire Disorder.

Unfortunately, low libido is just one of the negative side effects of low T for women as other side effects include, infertility, high body fat, dry hair, sadness, frustration, fatigue, depression and decreased self-confidence and self-worth.

And if you're worried about becoming too bulky from strength training, forget it. Unless your injecting steroids or bodybuilding with loads of unnatural supplements you simply will not become bulky like a man. This is due to the fact that men naturally produce more than three times the amount of Testosterone than women do.

The good news is, most of the key benefits Testosterone creates for men can also be found in females including:

- Maintenance and growth of bones
- Increases muscle mass
- Decreases body fat
- Lifts your libido or sex drive
- Helps support your cardiovascular health

Burns Fat And Helps You Lose Weight

Burning extra fat makes you lighter on your feet, builds your immune system against invaders like COVID-19, extends your life and makes you more attractive. Unlike traditional cardio, strength training causes you to continue burning more calories for up to 72 hours after the exercise is over through a process known as "after burn."

Turns back the clock

One study showed that strength training in the elderly reversed oxidative stress and returned 179 genes to their youthful level. In other words, it genetically turned back the clock about 10 years.[26] Strength training is also known to beneficially impact 10 biomarkers of aging, which are determinants of longevity and can extend your life.

Increases HGH

Human Growth Hormone is a sort of superpower of the hormone family. This is the stuff you had an abundance of as a teenager, which helped you heal a broken bone in half the time as an adult and if you're a dude, get a boner six times a day. It is without a doubt, one of your greatest sources of superpower and is responsible for the following awesomeness:

- Increases Testosterone production
- Improves immune function
- Increased exercise performance
- Better kidney function
- Stronger bones
- Younger, tighter skin
- Fat loss
- Higher energy levels and enhanced sexual performance
- Regrowth of heart, liver, spleen, kidneys, and other organs that shrink with age
- Greater heart output and lowered blood pressure
- Improved cholesterol profile
- Hair regrowth

Sadly, as you age, your ability to produce HGH decreases and by the time you start pushing 40 years old, your HGH levels will be around a third of what they were as a teenager.

Fortunately, there is really good news here and according to a study published by the International Journal of Sports Medicine in 1991, heavy resistance training can increase human growth hormone (HGH) in men and women from 200-700 percent.

Makes Your Bones Strong And Prevents Osteoporosis

It's a well-known fact that strength training can prevent and even reverse osteoporosis through its ability to build bone density. [27] And with strong bones you'll be much more likely to stay out of the wheelchair and active for the rest of your life.

Builds A Strong Heart

If you don't already know, heart disease is the #1 cause of death for both men and women. Thankfully, strength training works to build cardiovascular health by increasing blood circulation, lowering blood pressure and improving cholesterol levels. This was proven in one study when researchers compared the volume of blood being pumped into the heart from running versus leg presses. Leg presses won hands down. [28]

Prevents Diabetes

By controlling blood sugar and managing energy levels, strength training helps prevent diabetes and the crash and burn of too much sugar in your diet. While this is not an excuse to eat more sugar and carbs, it does help you deal with occasional hiccups in your diet – like your last birthday.

Increases Memory And Learning Abilities

We mentioned BDNF and its ability to build new brain cells earlier but it's worth repeating since diseases like Alzheimer's and other brain degenerative disorders are on the rise. Fortunately, strength training increases BDNF.

Improves Strength

While this is the most obvious of all the benefits, it's important to understand that muscle strength protects you from joint failure and organ failure. So if you have a skiing accident but you're knees are insulated with lots of muscle fibers from strength training, you'll be less likely to incur damage. Similarly, if your kidneys or heart fail for any reason but you have lots of muscle, this will delay organ failure and possibly even save your life.

Strength Training For Life - Bullet

Proofing Beliefs

"You have two choices, make excuses or make progress" - Tony Robbins

Whether you make excuses or make progress in strength training depends on your belief about it. And regardless of whether or not you're aware of any reluctance to strength training, it's important to look at your underlying belief about it and make absolutely sure nothing stands in the way of you and your island full of treasure.

To do this you'll need to answer four critical questions, which have been strategically crafted to shift your focus from disempowered to empowered and create a lifetime habit. In the personal development world, we call this process "neurological repatterning," which is really just a fancy phrase for changing beliefs.

Effectively, this process works to rewire your mindset and its associated beliefs to access more resourceful states, which then help you take more action and manifest your most sought after desires.

Time For Action

Below are four critical questions you'll need to answer in order to start the belief change process. If you're at all unsure about how to answer a question just reference the examples provided.

1) How did your old belief play out in a Circle of Results Model?

To assist you in identifying your old beliefs I've listed the most common limiting beliefs about strength training below. As you read them, be honest about which applies most accurately to your own circumstances and use them in the following exercise. If none apply, don't skip this exercise; instead, create your own.

I'm too old – Multiple studies conclude that no age is too old for strength training. And as mentioned earlier, strength training has been proven to turn back the clock by 10 years.

It's boring – Strength training may not be like hiking in Yosemite or skiing down the Swiss Alps but we can definitely take out the boring factor and enhance the awesomeness by adding music and mixing it up with different routines. Fortunately, in *Fired Up*, you'll never get bored because we use the synergy of Yoga, Strength Training and HIT and each discipline has multiple routines to choose from.

I don't want to be sore – Yes you can expect to be sore a few days after exercising for the first time or after not doing it for a while, but as your muscles get used to the movement they will get less and less sore each time. And here's the really good news: Since you'll be alternating with Yoga and HIT your muscles will be given more time to repair and you'll have the added synergy of Yoga to compliment healing. Rapid recovery can also be enhanced with proper nutrition so make sure you check out *The Power Diet* *if you don't already own it.*

I don't want to bulk up – Whether you do or don't want to bulk up, strength training in and of itself does NOT lead to bulk. The bulk comes from eating an irregular diet, loading up on supplements and following a bodybuilding exercise routine.

Fired Up is not a course on bodybuilding nor do I recommend anyone practice extreme exercise or overeating. These extreme practices can lead to injury, tax your mind and body, reduce your lifespan, and potentially lead to disease. In fact, a study published in the Journal of Exercise Rehabilitation in 2018 showed that the highest rate of injury for exercise disciplines came from bodybuilding and golf.[29]

Remember, our goal is optimal health and superhuman strength. If your goal is to get as huge as possible, it's important to think about what's behind this motivation and does is really serve yourself and the greater good of the world.

Circle of Results Model Example

Below is an example of a Circle of Results Model, which answers question #1 using an example from above. As you read it, take a note on how you can use this format to craft your own model.

1) What did you pretend to believe which when realized would make this disempowered belief go away forever?

B – I pretended to believe that my self-worth was determined by how much others approved of me. I pretended to believe that unlike others, I wasn't worthy of having a strong and fit body, that my friends, family, and others who told me I was weak and worthless were right. I use to believe working out would always be painful and that I'd always be judged as being weak so I never did it.

T – I used to think, "Oh my God I'm going to look like a fool, everyone will laugh at me and I'll be sore for a week."

E – I felt stressed, anxious and apprehensive at just the thought of working out.

A – Instead of working out I would just revert to food, TV and my couch for comfort.

R – I became weak, overweight and depressed from my lack of activity.

Write down your "Old Belief" in a Circle of Results Model.

2) What are the problems created by your old belief?

Describe the problems your old belief created – i.e., how much time was wasted, any bad habits you developed, how did you suffer, how did it make you feel?

For example: I wasted 100's of hours on the couch watching TV instead of getting *Fired Up* and pursuing my passions. I would sit down and eat a gallon of ice cream while binge watching Netflix from the time I got home until the time I went to bed. I didn't sleep well and suffered from insomnia. I stopped respecting myself and so did the people around me. To feel better I would just distract myself with more vices and create even more pain. I felt stuck, depressed and hopeless.

Write Down The Problems Created by Your Old Belief

____

3) What are the benefits of your problem?

If there were a benefit to having this problem what would it be? Is there something that your unconscious mind wants you to understand that if you understood it would make the problem disappear?

For example: I realized that the reason people judged me for being weak had nothing to do with me. These people were insecure and needed to put others down in order to feel good about themselves. I also realized that I was just making excuses, doubting myself and postponing my dreams. I learned that failure from the past doesn't mean failure in the future. This new perspective allowed me to step my game up, take action and start building myself with *The Power Diet* and the *Fired Up* program.

Write Down The Benefits Of Your Problem

____

New Belief Change Declaration #1 – Strength Training Is Powerful

Now its time to declare your new belief by writing it down in a Circle of Results Model and then focus on it daily.

4) **How will your "New Belief" play out in a Circle of Results Model?**

Example:

B – I believe the fear of embarrassment and rejection is just a story, an excuse to remain stuck. I also believe in myself without the need for approval from others. I believe strength training makes me more sexually potent, strong and powerful so I can stand up for myself, take action, contribute more to society and live my life purpose. It's a privilege, which helps me see the world much more clearly.

T – I think someone is judging, how sad, they must be insecure and dissatisfied with themselves. I think, I can't wait to get *Fired Up*; nothing makes me feel so alive and full of power.   I think, I'm really working on myself and moving forward, nothing can stop me now!

E – I feel deeply satisfied and empowered like nothing can take away my joy and confidence. I feel compassion for those who need to criticize others, as I know they're doing the best with what they got. I feel excited about the future because I know every day I just keep getting stronger.

A – I read *Fired Up* and *The Power Diet* then implement all the strategies.

R – Within 30 days of starting the *Fired Up* program I start to see noticeable changes in my mind and body. I feel stronger and more powerful. People start to ask: "What's different about you?" They respect me more and want what I have. This gives me more confidence to take more action and pursue my passions. The extra energy and confidence lead to a new side business consulting for business owners and I've attracted a new girlfriend who spends the night at my house 5 nights a week.

Now write down a Circle of Results Model using your "New Belief":

New Belief: What do you declare as your new belief? Make sure you use Pain, Pleasure and Purpose as well as the Master Mindsets that feel most empowering to you.

____

Thought: Describe the thoughts you'll have after you've embedded this new belief.

____

Emotion: Describe how you will feel once this new belief is part of your permanent mindset.

____

Action: What have you been unwilling to do in order to keep this problem? Describe the action you will take which will lead to a new habit.

____

____

Result: How do you know for sure that your old belief is no longer a problem for you? Visualize your new outcome in detail – i.e., where will you be, who will be with you, any new habits created from the action, how will you feel?

____

Take Action

Congratulations you've just created a new empowered belief about strength training. Just keep in mind, in order to embed this belief deep into your subconscious and make it a more permanent part of your roots, you'll need to repeat it to yourself daily for 60-90 days, which will create a long-term habit.

What I recommend is you write your Circle of Results Model down in your smartphone on a notepad.

Next, open your electronic calendar and write a reminder that repeats every day for the next 90 days. All you have to do is read the note when that reminder pops up, it's really that simple.

To make it even more effective, try to memorize it and repeat it out loud to yourself.

Last but definitely not least, make absolutely sure you tell a friend or family member about your new belief and how you are committed to keeping it. This is absolutely crucial as studies show telling others about a goal helps you stay accountable and committed to upholding that belief.

For example, in one study, researchers found that you have a 65% chance of completing a goal if you commit to someone. Additionally, if you have a specific accountability appointment with a person you've committed, you will increase your chance of success by up to 95%.[30]

Take action on this and do not hesitate. If you can do this, I guarantee you'll thank me later when your new superhuman powers start appearing from out of nowhere.

The Exercises

Now that you've got your roots solidified in concrete beliefs that motivate and sustain you through the tough times, it's time to get down and dirty with the nuts and bolts of strength training. Let's start with the first and most important question:

What Are The Best Exercises For Maximum Impact?

To be clear, while you'll be building superhuman power and a body that is both incredibly strong and flexible, this is not a bodybuilding course that requires two hours in the gym, 15 different exercises and 50 sets 5 days a week.

Instead, we'll take the best and most impactful exercises from the strength training canon and add them to our synergy of *Fired Up* power boosters.

To do this, we're going to be focusing primarily on movements called "Compound Exercises," which activate the maximum amount of muscle volume per movement.

In other words, we'll use exercises that engage as many large muscles at one time as possible. The beauty of compound exercises is that they help you build superhuman power in three primary ways:

1) **Saves Time** – By training multiple muscles at once you don't have to spend hours in the gym doing isolation exercises. This frees up time to work on your passions and spend time doing the things you love most.

2) **Builds More Muscle Faster** – Compound exercises allow you to lift heavier weights than isolation exercises, which progressively overloads your muscles and leads to faster muscle growth.

3) **Boosts Testosterone and Human Growth Hormone** – Since the total amount of muscle involved in your workout is directly related to the amount of anabolic hormones created, compound exercises significantly boost testosterone and growth hormone levels far beyond isolation exercises and studies prove this.[31] For example, the rack squat engages over 200 different muscles and I'll show you a variation of chin-ups, which engage your pecks, shoulders, triceps, biceps, abs, quads and hamstrings all simultaneously.

But remember, this isn't about becoming a beer can crushing meathead. Instead, our goal is to work towards a broad range of superhuman powers, which means in addition to those compound exercises we'll also focus on a few key "Isolation Exercises," which allow you to function closer to 100% capacity in daily life.

It's all well and good to be able to bench press 300 pounds, but if you can't lift your arm over your head because your internal and external rotator cuff muscles (supraspinatus, infraspinatus, teres minor, and subscapularis) are weak, injured or out of balance you may need to get a ladder to simply reach the coffee mug from the cupboard.

If you have yet to injure a joint like hips, knees, ankles or shoulders I can pretty much guarantee without working on isolation exercises, stretching and getting rid of the inflammation in your diet you will eventually encounter a major problem. If you're at all skeptical consider the fact that in the year 2017, there were approximately 1.6 million hip and knee replacements performed in the United States alone.[32]

The problem occurs when muscles, whose normal function is to stabilize and protect joints, are not exercised, overstressed or out of balance. In this case, you not only become more vulnerable to injury but your daily movements become restricted.

Fortunately, I've been involved in sports my whole life and have experienced the process of rehabilitation from some major joint injuries which I mentioned earlier. But you don't need to be an athlete to tear ligaments and cartilage. I've had clients tear ligaments just walking up the stairs or getting out of their car.

So while we'll focus primarily on compound exercises, we'll also focus on isolation exercises that help strengthen and stabilize your joints. This will essentially bulletproof your joints against future injury and increase your mobility so you can function more efficiently in daily life.

First, let's talk about those compound exercises.

The 3 Types Of Compound Exercise

Strength Training is not rocket science. When it comes to compound exercises there are only three primary categories you need to remember - push, pull and legs.

The Three Primary Exercises Are Push, Pull & Legs

The Six Muscle Groups

While push, pull and legs are the broader categories of strength training; we'll need to focus on some specific muscle groups within those categories to design a workout that leads to your ideal body with maximum power. Specifically, here are your six master muscle groups we'll be building:

1) **Chest -** Your chest is made up primarily from the sternocostal head of your pecs, which is emphasized in the flat bench press, while the smaller clavicular head is emphasized in the incline bench press. Together, the flat and incline bench press

will develop maximum size pecs and gorilla-like power in your chest.

2) **Shoulders -** Your shoulder consists of several muscles, the three most prominent are the deltoids: Anterior (front) deltoid Lateral (side) deltoid Posterior (rear) deltoid. We'll be engaging these muscles in just about every exercise that uses your upper body.

3) **Back -** Your back has a multitude of muscles including the Trapezius, Rhomboids, Latissimus dorsi, Erector spinae, Teres major, Teres minor and Infraspinatus. As one of the most undertrained groups of muscles, your back is responsible for pulling your upper arms toward your torso and stabilizing your shoulder blades, neck, and spine (amongst other things). Neglecting these key muscles could lead to poor posture and shoulder injury from an imbalance between your "push" and "pull" muscles. For this reason, we'll focus just as much time on your back as your chest and shoulders.

4) **Arms -** The primary arm muscles include your biceps, triceps and forearms.

5) **Legs & Glutes -** The primary leg muscles we'll be focusing on are your Quadriceps (quads) Hamstrings and Calves. And while your glutes are not officially part of your legs they are engaged and

strengthened in all of our compound leg exercises so we'll include them here to keep it simple. This includes the gluteus maximus, gluteus medius and gluteus minimus, which originate from your ilium and sacrum and insert on your femur bone. These hard working muscles are critical for daily function and stabilize your femur (thighbone) in your hip socket, rotate your femur internally and externally, and draw your leg back so you can stand and walk. Kind of important don't you think?

6) **Core -** Your core includes the rectus abdominis, transverse abdominis, and internal and external obliques. We'll talk in detail about the critical nature of these muscles in our isolation exercises shortly.

Combining Muscle Groups Into Optimal Compound Exercises

Now is the fun part, where we get to see which exercises combine those six muscle groups and give us maximum power using the most optimal compound exercises.

Push Exercises (chest, shoulders, forearms, back and triceps)

- Barbell Bench Press (Incline and Flat)
- Dumbbell Bench Press (Incline and Flat)

- Push Ups (Spiderman, Superman, regular)
- Dips
- Triceps Pushdown
- Dumbbell Overhead (Military) Press
- Barbell Overhead (Military) Press

Pull (biceps, shoulders, forearms and back)

- Pull-Up
- Chin-Up
- Seated Rows
- Lat Pulldown (Wide- and Close-Grip)

Legs (quadriceps, hamstrings, glutes and calves)

- Barbell Squat
- Reverse Barbell Lunge
- Bulgarian Split Lunge
- Deadlift
- Leg Press

How Many Compound Exercises Should I Do Per Workout?

To get the most out of your workout I recommend sticking to 3-6 compound exercises per workout session. There are three primary reasons for this including:

- Allows proper time for recovery

- Allows you to work all major muscle groups
- Works to create synergy between HIIT and Yoga

Do 3-6 Compound Exercises Per Workout

The Isolation Exercises

While there are literally dozens of isolation exercises, similar to compound exercises we'll be focusing on a few of the most important ones, which function to bulletproof the most common problem areas like your back, hips and knees.

Just keep in mind, very few if any "isolation" exercises only focus on one muscle. This is term is used quite loosely since in reality most isolation exercises simply "emphasize" a targeted muscle while engaging other muscles in the surrounding area. To keep it simple, we'll call these isolation exercises.

For example, if you have challenges with back problems, there's a good chance that your abdominal muscles are weak and by strengthening them you may be able to reduce or eliminate those problems.

And let's not forget the powerful synergy of yoga from the *Fired Up* program, which, interestingly enough, is also the primary form of exercise recommended by doctors to fix back pain.

Core Strength & Stability

The importance of strengthening your core (abdominal muscles) cannot be underestimated and will be addressed in all three of our synergistic disciplines - yoga, HIIT and strength training. And while various compound exercises do address the sought after six-pack abs, research shows they don't involve much of the "show" muscles of the rectus abdominis, transverse abdominis, and external obliques to actually give you a six-pack.[33]

Accordingly, you'll need to do some targeted core work as well as shed unnecessary fat using an advance diet program like *The Power Diet* if you really want to get those six-pack abs.

And more importantly, since most people tend to avoid doing core work, you'll need to create a strong belief that core work brings immense benefits to your daily life in order to actually commit to doing it and seeing long-term results.

To help you in your efforts I've broken down the muscles and how they enhance and make your daily life more enjoyable with less pain. Notice how the following four muscles play into your own personal circumstances and feel free to go back and change your Circle of Results Model if you struggle with core work.

- **Your Six Pack** – Your six pack is technically called the "rectus abdominis," which is the long, flat muscle that extends vertically between your pubis and your fifth, sixth, and seventh ribs. Your six-pack helps you flex your spinal column so you can bend over and pick up that bag of groceries. It also helps with side bending motions and stabilizing your trunk when you need to use your legs and arms to put that bag in your car.

- **The V** – Technically called "external oblique muscles," this pair of muscles is located on each side of your rectus abdominis and runs diagonally downward and inward from your lower ribs to your pelvis, forming the letter V. These muscles allow for flexion of your spine so you can bend over and tie your shoes as well as rotate your torso so you can turn and see the driver that almost hit you on the freeway.

- **The V Below The V** - Your "internal oblique" muscles are a pair of deep muscles that are just below the external oblique muscles and reinforce the external obliques by helping you flex your spinal column, bend sideways and swing a golf club with just enough power to drive it 300 yards and win the day.

- **The Weight Belt** – Your "transversus abdominis" muscle wraps around your torso from front to back and from your ribs to your pelvis. The muscle fibers of the transversus abdominis run horizontally, similar to a weight belt, and helps stabilize your spine so you can rearrange the chairs when guests come over or throw your woman (or man) on the bed without breaking your back.

Knee Strength & Stability

Similar to your stomach muscles, your inner thigh muscles, also known as the five adductor muscles
(pectineus, gracilis, adductor
longus, adductor brevis, and adductor magnus) together, function to provide stability and injury prevention for your knees, hips, and lower back (to name a few).

This group of muscles creates internal rotation, which counterbalances the external rotation from your outer thighs and glutes. Essentially, this helps your knees track properly and perform compound exercises, like squats and lunges. All five adductor muscles attach to your pelvis, which means weak inner thighs could create poor balance and send you tumbling as you try to navigate a simple staircase.

While the adductors pull your leg inward, your abductor muscles in your hips pull your legs away from the midline of your body. Basically, every time you step to the side, get in the car or get out of bed, you're using your abductors. If you have underdeveloped or neglected abductors you'll most likely feel vulnerable in your knee joints and struggle with the basics like standing, walking and running with ease.

Shoulder Strength & Stability

Last but not least, your shoulders are also made up of a group of muscles starting with the primary muscle - the deltoid. As the largest shoulder muscle covering of your glenohumeral joint, your deltoids have different muscle fibers that are responsible for different actions, like raising your arm when you need to clutch the steering wheel and get off the freeway before you miss your exit.

The strength of your deltoid is also responsible for preventing joint dislocation when you're carrying that big heavy luggage bag that weighs 100 pounds and doesn't want to squeeze into the trunk.

But perhaps the most neglected of all is the rotator cuff. As a group of muscles and tendons surrounding your shoulder joint, the rotator cuff's job is to keep the head of your upper arm bone firmly within the shallow socket of your shoulder.

Injuries to the rotator cuff are quite common. I mentioned my struggles earlier but this happens to anyone who is either aging or does a lot of repetitive motion like artists, musicians, painters, carpenters, and people who play baseball or tennis. Without strength and agility in your rotator cuff you may find yourself up all night counting sheep because it's too painful to sleep on your side (assuming you're a side sleeper).

Fortunately, we'll be addressing the deltoid and the four muscles in your rotator cuff (supraspinatus, infraspinatus, teres minor, and subscapularis) so you can bulletproof your shoulders as well as your knees.

The Biceps Brachii

The biceps brachii (AKA biceps) is a double-headed muscle involved in the movement of your elbow and shoulder. The short head of each biceps brachii originates at the top of your scapula while the long head originates just above your shoulder joint. Both heads are joined at your elbow and help control the motion of your shoulder and your elbow when lifting that bag of groceries or that six-pack of beer (depending on the day of the week).

The Isolation Exercises

Now that you have a basic understanding of the critical functions of these muscle groups, let's move on to the stabilizing exercises, which bulletproof these areas.

While all of these groups will be addressed to a certain degree with our compound exercises, the following exercises will isolate, emphasize and target specific muscles that support the most vulnerable areas.

Core (all 4 abdominal muscles)

- Hanging Knee Raise
- Captain's Chair Leg Raise
- Lying Leg Raise
- Weighted Sit-Up
- Plank
- Abdominal Rollout
- Cross Leg Taps
- Butterfly Crunches

Knees & Hip Joints (calves, quads, hams, glutes, adductor & abductor muscles)

While there are several great strength training exercises to insulate and protect these critical joints, leg extensions are not one of them. The problem with leg extension machines is that they put a tremendous amount of pressure on your knee joints, which is simply not worth the risk of injury. As such, make sure you avoid the leg extension machine (aka knee extension).

Instead, in the *Fired Up* program, we'll be using primarily compound exercises like the squat and the following isolation exercises to bulletproof your knees and hips.

- Adductor Exercises (machine, dumbbell or resistance bands)
  Dumbbell goblet adductor side lunge, side lunge with eagle arms

- Abductors (machine or resistance bands)
  Sidestep with hip band ladder, lateral leg lifts

- Split lunge & Side Lunge with or without dumbbells

Shoulders Joints (deltoids and all 4 rotator cuff muscles)

- Internal and external rotation (resistance bands, cables or free weights)
- Lateral, frontal, angled arm raises (resistance bands, cables or free weights)

Biceps (biceps and forearms)

- E-Z Bar Curl
- Alternating Dumbbell Curl
- Dumbbell Hammer Curl

How Many Isolation Exercises Should I Do Per Workout?

I recommend sticking to 2-4 isolation exercises per workout session. The three primary reasons for this are the same as compound exercises including:

- Allows proper time for recovery.
- Allows you to work stabilizer muscles, which protect key joints and spine.
- Works to create synergy between HIIT and Yoga.

Do 2-4 isolation exercises per workout session

How Many Reps Should I Do?

Remember that we are trying to build maximum testosterone, strength and muscle, which means we need to conform to a specific rep range and intensity.

First, for those who are not already familiar with strength training lingo, let's go over a little of the terminology.

"Rep" is simply shorthand for "repetition," which represents a single movement of lifting some type of weight upwards then lowering it down.

"Set" is a fixed number of reps done consecutively without stopping.

In *Fired Up* we're going to shoot for 8-15 reps per set on isolation exercises and 4–8 reps per set on compound exercises.

First, let's talk about compound exercises. In this case, the amount of weight you lift 4-8 times should equate to around 80% of your 1 rep max (the maximum weight you can lift the weight 1 time).

Your goal is to reach positive failure within that 4-8 rep range. This is the point where you cannot do any more reps and will be referred to as a **"Hard Set"** throughout this training.

Why 4-8? According to studies, research shows that this rep range is highly effective for gaining muscle and strength.[34] Additionally, this range proves to be heavy enough to create maximum muscle and strength but not so heavy that it becomes dangerous or uncontrollable.

In a meta-analysis (in-depth examination of multiple studies) scientists at Lehman College and Victoria University reviewed 21 studies that compared training with heavier weights (60-plus percent of one-rep max) and lower reps versus lighter weights (less than 60 percent of one-rep max) and higher reps.

The scientists discovered that both strategies caused similar amounts of muscle growth, but training with heavier weights caused greater increases in strength.

Researchers also noted that training with lighter weights only resulted in significant muscle growth when sets were taken to, or close to, positive muscle failure (the point where you can't do any more reps).[35]

Now let's talk about those isolation exercises. If you're wondering why you should be doing more reps for isolation exercises here are two good reasons.

First off, your smaller muscles like biceps and triceps are used individually for everyday movements like pushing and pulling and by training them for endurance, rather than power, you become more functional.

Second, for compound exercises that create strength and power like squats, it's okay to go heavy for 4-6 reps because the load is distributed across your joints (ankles, knees, hips, and spine, etc.). In contrast, isolation exercises put all the strain on one area, which can overload the joint for the benefit of the muscle and put you at a higher risk for injury. Increasing your reps forces you to lift less weight and in the process protects your joints.   So remember this:

- **Compound Exercises Reps** **4-8**

- **Isolation Exercises Reps** **8-15**

No Gym No Weights = More Reps

While 4-8 reps may be ideal for maximum strength gains, if you can do more than 8 reps of a particular exercise (Main muscle groups or isolation exercises) and don't belong to a gym, don't have access to one or simply don't want to go to one, this range can increase to whatever number of reps it takes to get to positive failure. As you just learned from the study mentioned above, this strategy works almost as well as 4-8 reps with just a slight compromise in strength gain.

Shortly, we'll talk about changing the tempo of the rep and staying within your rep range without having to add weight, but for now just know that if you can do more than 8 reps of a particular exercise and the gym is not an option, keep going until you reach positive failure whether that's 10, 15 or 20 reps!

The Double Progression Model

If you do have access to the gym and use weights to strength train, we'll be employing the use of one of the most time-tested strategies available most commonly referred to as: "The Double Progression Model."

Essentially, with this model, your goal is to add weight once you can consistently come within 1-2 reps (6-8) of the top of your rep range. Then, once you add weight, if you can consistently lift it 4 reps or more, you'll keep working with that weight until once again you progress to within 1-2 reps (6-8) of the top of your rep range.

This model will help you progress and breakthrough plateaus, which may have seemed impossible to surmount. Essentially, your goal is to increase your reps, then "cash in" that progress to increase your total volume of weight lifted. Hence, "double progression."

For example, let's say you're bench pressing 4-8 reps, and on the first hard set of your workout you manage push 150 pounds 8 times. Then, on your second set, you get 6 reps in. Based on the *Fired Up* protocol, you've just demonstrated consistently pushing within 1-2 reps of your upper range, which means its time to increase the weight.

The next set you make the total volume 155-160 pounds by adding 5-10 pounds and do at least 4 reps. Congratulations! You've just progressed!

Just remember, in order to make double progression work you must end each of your hard sets at least one or two reps shy of positive failure (the point where you can't do anymore reps safely).

CAUTION!

Pushing, pulling or lifting to full technical failure could put you at risk for injury.

To elucidate this pitfall we need to look no further than the dude in the gym who you might have encountered on TV or perhaps up close and personal. He seemed out of control, didn't know what he was doing or maybe he just fell prey to "Overkill" and the lesser ego. Either way, he somehow managed to find himself under a barbell screaming at the top of his lungs to complete that one last rep but just couldn't find the strength to do so, at which point the weight collapsed on him or someone had to save him.

Sadly, this scenario places the lifter at a high risk of injury and was demonstrated by a study that showed how pushing to technical failure leads to a breakdown if form, potential injury and is not necessary for muscle and strength gain.[36]

Don't be one of those dudes! Make sure your last rep is under your control (aka positive failure), especially if you are lifting free weights without a spotter.

Rep Tempo - How Fast Or Slow Should Your Reps Be?

How fast or slow you lift and lower weight is referred to as "Rep tempo" and is considered another major area of heated debate in the weight lifting world. So before we move on I'd like to issue a word of caution. Believing there is only one way will limit your options and is subject to one of our primary pitfalls mentioned at the beginning of *Fired Up* - The "One Way Trap."

For example, those who advocate for a slow tempo (AKA Super Slow Strength Training) often say that "muscles don't know weight, only tension," and the more tension they're subjected to, the more the potential for workload and muscle gain.   So by simply slowing down the movement (decreasing the tempo), you create more tension by extending the time under load.

In contrast, those who advocate faster tempo argue that total reps performed with a given muscle group over time is a major factor in muscle gain and that super slow training results in less work done, which reduces the muscle and   strength-building potential of the exercise, which is scientifically valid.[37]

But after reviewing the studies in detail it turns out that both slow and fast tempo can work to your advantage.

Ironically, in one experiment, researchers found that a slower tempo of the bench press actually created greater strength gains than fast tempo (9.1% vs. 8.6% respectively). Yet when it came to the squat, the faster tempo beat out slower tempo by almost double (6.8% vs. 3.6% respectively).[38]

Evening out the playing field between fast and slow tempo was demonstrated by another study published in *Medicine & Science* in *Sports & Exercise,* which concluded that doing faster reps gives you 11% more strength gain than slow tempo but only when sets were restricted to 1 set. In contrast, when participants of the study (both slow and fast tempo) were compared for strength gains after 3 sets the results did not show a statistical difference worth mentioning.

The good news is that in *Fired Up* you'll have the option of training with or without weights using either slow or fast tempo, depending on your circumstances.

Rep Tempo For Super Slow Strength Training

"Super Slow Strength Training" is a variation of Strength Training, which can be considered HIIT with all its accompanying benefits.   Research from fitness experts, Dr. Doug McGuff and Phil Campbell have shown how a normal weight training routine can become a high intensity routine by simply slowing it down.   Effectively, by doing this you activate both your aerobic and anaerobic systems, which qualifies this workout as both Strength Training and HIIT.

The good news is that you can perform the super-slow technique with many of the strength training exercises already discussed such as hand weights, resistance machines, bodyweight exercises, or resistance bands.

The beauty of this routine is that you only need about 12 minutes of Super-Slow type strength training once a week to achieve the same growth hormone production as you would from 20 minutes of Peak Fitness sprints. The key to making it work is intensity. The intensity needs to be high enough that you reach muscle fatigue.

Interestingly enough, when the intensity is high, you can also decrease the frequency of your exercise. In fact, in order to continue to be productive, the higher your fitness level, the more you can decrease the frequency without losing benefits. This is because, as a beginner, you can exercise three times a week and not put much stress on your system. But once your strength and endurance improve, each exercise session is placing an increasingly greater amount of stress on your body (as long as you keep pushing yourself to the max). At that point, you'll want to reduce the frequency of your sessions to give your body enough time to recover in between workouts.

How To Do Super Slow Strength Training

I recommend keeping it simple and using four or five basic compound movements for your super-slow exercise sets. Compound movements are movements that require the coordination of several muscle groups. For example, squats, chest presses, and compound rows.

Start by lifting, pushing or pulling the weight slowly and gradually for 4-8 seconds then lower it for another 4-8 seconds. Also, when pushing, stop about 10 to 15 degrees before your limb is fully straightened and then smoothly reverse direction. Repeat this until exhaustion, which should be around 4-8 reps (see _Fired Up_ videos for clarity).

Once you reach exhaustion, don't try to heave or jerk the weight to get one last repetition in. Instead, just keep trying to produce the movement, even if it's not "going" anywhere, for another five seconds or so. If you're using the appropriate amount of weight or resistance, you'll be able to perform four to eight reps.

Once you finish each set, immediately switch to the next exercise for the next target muscle group and try to get another 4-8 reps in. The amount of sets can vary but shoot for a minimum of 12 minutes and try not to go past 30 minutes or you could overstrain yourself.

If you do not have weights and can't add enough weight to stay within the 4-8 rep range you can simply slow down your movement, which will make each rep more difficult and get you closer to your ideal rep range. While this won't give you quite the strength gains as a faster tempo with more weight, it will allow you to increase your time under load and overall workload, which will help you build more strength and muscle.

Just remember, Super Slow tempo is one of several options. As mentioned earlier in the studies, you can still get amazing benefits by doing as many reps as it takes to get to positive failure whether that be 10, 15 or 20 reps.

Rep Tempo For Fast Strength Training

If you do have access to weights or a gym faster tempo will allow you to build more strength. So what is faster tempo?

Shoot for a "1–1" rep tempo; this would mean when you push, pull or lift weight it should take about one second, followed by a one-second lowering of the weight. According to scientists at the University of Sydney, this rep tempo has been proven to help gain 11% more strength on the bench press than with slow training.[39]

How Many Sets Per Exercise Should I Do?

As another area of heated debate, which is also subject to the "One Way" pitfall, is the amount of sets you do per exercise. Some say all you need is 1 set, while others claim you need up to 6 sets to create maximum strength, muscle and power. Fortunately, studies suggest you get more bang for your buck by doing a moderate amount of sets.

For example, according to a landmark study in 1998, researchers found that there was no significant difference in strength or muscle mass as a result of single versus multiple sets.[40] While this study revealed some interesting insights a more recent study in 2002 concluded that trained exercisers get more strength gains out of multi-set training.[41]

Additional studies have bolstered the claims of multiple sets, most importantly a 2009 study, which found that 2-3 sets per exercise were associated with a 46 percent greater strength gain than one set in both trained and untrained subjects.[42]

And finally, to put this debate to rest, a 2010 study showed a similar gain in muscle growth in trained and untrained subjects who completed multiple sets.[43]

In conclusion, based on the prevailing studies, by doing multiple sets you will gain more strength but not necessarily more muscle.

So how many sets are best?

This depends on your ability level and time restrictions. While you're not going to get all the strength gains of multiple sets, if you're short on time or just starting out, one set could be just enough.

1 Set Per Exercise Could Be Just Enough

For example, let's say you are short on time or just starting out on the *Fired Up* program and building your way up (setting your ego aside). You could do a full body routine with just 1 set of the following 8 exercises and be done in 15 minutes:

1) Pull-Ups
2) Chin-Ups
3) Push-Ups Or Bench Press
4) Dips
5) Squats
6) Hanging Knee Raises
7) Lateral Raise
8) Front Raise

2-3 Sets Per Exercise Is Ideal

Now assuming you have a good 30 minutes or more you can boost testosterone, strength and lean muscle mass to superhuman levels with 2-3 sets per exercise for both your compound and isolation movements.

How Many Sets Per Workout Should I Do?

Now that you have an optimal range of sets per exercise, let's talk about the optimal number of sets per workout. Ideally, you'll shoot for a range of 8-16 total sets per workout.

1 Set Workout

As just mentioned, if you're doing 1 set per exercise, an 8 set minimum would give you a quick full body blast, which should take no longer than 15 minutes including rest.

2-3 Set Workout

If you have 30 minutes or more try pushing to a minimum of 8 total sets and up to 16. For example, let's say you do 2 sets of 3 compound exercises and 2 sets of 3 isolation exercises. This would equal 4-8 reps of 12 total sets as follows:

Pull-Ups 4-8 reps x 2 sets
Chin-Ups 4-8 reps x 2 sets
Spiderman Pushups or Bench Press 4-8 reps x 2 sets
Hanging Knee Raises 8-15 reps x 2 sets
Lateral Arm Raises 8-15 reps x 2 sets
Front Arm Raises 8-15 reps x 2 sets

____

6 x 2 = 12 sets

Alternatively, if you're feeling strong, kick it up a notch with 3 sets of 4 compound exercises and 2 sets of 2 isolation exercises. In this scenario, you would do 4-8 reps multiplied x 16 sets. Here's an example:

Pull-Ups 4-8 reps x 3 sets
Chin-Ups 4-8 reps x 3 sets
Squats 4-8 reps x 3 sets
Spiderman Pushups or Bench Press 4-8 reps x 3 sets
Hanging Knee Raises 8-15 reps x 2 sets
Adductor Exercises 8-15 reps x 2 sets

$$(3 \times 4) + (2 \times 2) = 16$$

As you can see, when it comes to creating a workout routine, there are a multitude of options to choose from. So while the *Fired Up* program will give you several suggested routines, I highly encourage you to explore and test different routines that may work better for your circumstances.

That being said, in the interest of safety and injury prevention it's also important you review the videos that come with the *Fired Up* program for proper form and detailed instruction.

How Much Should I Rest Between Sets?

It is important to understand that as you work out you are breaking down muscle fiber, which means you'll need to allow ample time for rest and repair.

So how much time should you rest between sets?

Rest 2-3 Minutes Between Sets

Most studies prove the sweet spot is between 2 – 3 minutes, including a study at the Federal University of Parana, Brazil where researchers found that when people performed the bench press and squat with two-minute rest intervals, they were able to perform significantly more reps per workout than when rest intervals were shortened in 15-second increments (1:45, 1:30, 1:15, and so forth).[44]

What's significant about this finding is that studies also show the total amount of reps you perform over time is a major factor in muscle growth.[45]

In another study conducted by scientists at the State University of Rio de Janeiro researchers found that when training with loads between 50% and 90% of one repetition maximum, 3-5 minutes' rest between sets allowed for greater repetitions over multiple sets as well as greater increases in absolute strength, due to higher intensities and volumes of training. It should be noted that this study contrasted 3 or 5 minutes versus 1 minute of rest between sets.[46]

Similar findings were demonstrated in a study conducted by scientists at Eastern Illinois University where researchers demonstrated large squat strength gains could be achieved with a minimum of 2 minutes' rest between sets, and little additional gains are derived from resting more than 4 minutes between sets.[47]

As you can see, the sweet spot is around 2-3 minutes but unlike most trainers who will tell you to take a break and do nothing for 2-3 minutes, in Fired Up you'll be using this time to maximize your superhuman powers with isolation exercises as well as incorporating the synergy of Yoga, which will keep you occupied, energized and protected from injury. By watching the videos from the Fired

Up Video Program this will become much more clear.

To get a 25% discount on the Fired Up Video Program just use discount code: "Firedup-25-off-readers-only" and follow the link below:

https://chadscottcoaching.com/fired-up-lifetime/

How Much Should I Rest Between Workouts?

Although our goal of this program is to literally get you Fired Up so you can do things you never thought possible there is a point where too much Fire can lead to a burnt forest that may not ever recover. This could be one of the most dangerous pitfalls of not just strength training but all forms of exercise including HIIT and YOGA. Of course this relates back to our "Overkill" trap, so pay close attention here.

Many people who start getting benefits from strength training tend to think that if they just do more of the same thing the benefits will just keep multiplying. Sadly, this strategy is set up to fail.

Basically, without getting too scientific, it's important to understand that similar to a wound, when you workout, you are tearing down muscle fiber, which needs time to rest, recover, and build more muscle tissue than you had before.   This process is called *supercompensation* (you compensate a little to get a lot more).

When you strength train, you are not increasing the amount of muscle fibers you have; instead, you are increasing the size and overall mass of the fibers you already have, which is called hypertrophy.

While you've most likely heard of "anabolic" as in anabolic steroids, which builds muscles to monstrous proportions, you may not have heard of "catabolic," which is the process of breaking muscle fiber down.

While both of these processes are crucial for strength and muscle development if for any reason you're wondering about or considering taking anabolic steroids to leapfrog your way to the top, I can say first hand that you'll most likely regret that decision.

When I was playing D1 college football at San Diego State University, I broke my sternal clavicular joint when I was blindsided by a 260-pound Samoan linebacker as I jumped up to catch a pass. The pressure to recover quickly and get back on the field was so great that I was willing to do anything.

Interestingly enough, it just so happened that another linebacker friend of mine was pedaling steroids to about 20% of the entire team.

After caving in to pressure and completing one cycle of jamming painful needles full of anabolic steroids into my ass, I saw a major leap in strength and muscle growth. Unfortunately, it did not do anything for my injury and the side effects of emotional turbulence and a massive outbreak of acne made it simply unsustainable.

The good news is that with the *Fired Up* program you won't need anabolic steroids to get the most out of the anabolic phase.

In regards to the catabolic phase of working out, it is critical that you understand that by continuing to do the same exercise, without time for proper recovery, you are basically digging a deeper wound, which could actually set you up for a major injury. And while it may seem logical to attribute most injuries in strength training to overly intense workouts, studies show the real reason to be inadequate recovery time. [48]

Because of this, how frequently you do a particular exercise will always depend on how long it takes for that wound to heal itself and complete the anabolic phase of rebuilding. More specifically, your frequency will depend on two primary factors and four secondary factors as follows:

The 2 Primary Factors That Determine Rest Period

1) **Volume** – The volume represents how much weight you've lifted during the course of a workout.

2) **Intensity** – The intensity represents how many reps and sets you do during the course of a workout.

Studies confirm, the higher the volume and intensity of a workout the more muscle fiber is broken down (the deeper the wound) and the longer you'll need to wait until you exercise the same muscles.[49]

If for instance, you choose to do 1 hard set of pull-ups and chin-ups, the intensity and volume will be low enough to repeat these exercises 3 times a week on Monday, Wednesday and Friday. But if you do 3 hard sets of pull-ups and chin-ups the intensity and volume will be too much to repeat these exercises 3 times a week on Monday, Wednesday and Friday.

As a general rule of thumb, depending on volume and intensity, I recommend the following:

Train Major Muscle Groups 1-3 Times Per Week

We'll go into detail on exact recommendations shortly, just know that if you're feeling weak during a workout, like you can not lift as much as you could before, then you most likely need more rest. The bottom line here is this:

Listen To The Warning Signals From Your Body!

And don't be afraid to take more than 7 days of rest or more from a particular exercise and associated muscle group. Furthermore, depending on your circumstances, you may need 10, 14 or 21 days off a particular exercise to fully recover the muscles associated with that exercise. And remember, you're not going to be twiddling your thumbs during this rest period, you'll be engaging in the other elements of *Fired Up*, Yoga and HIIT, which will help you create the synergy of superhuman power.

The 4 Secondary Factors That Determine Rest Period

There are, of course, other factors, which may delay the process of recovery and stunt the anabolic process of rebuilding muscle, so let's examine four of the most common circumstances that could affect your performance.

1) **You're Just Getting Started** – If you've never done strength training or haven't done it for several months, your rest periods may be shorter than if you had been training consistently. If this is you, chances are you'll see significant strength gains within the first 3-6 months, at which point your gains will begin to slow down. This is widely known in lifting circles as the honeymoon phase because those big gains will eventually wear off. Don't be alarmed if this happens, just stick with the program and you'll be guided with solutions that will help overcome any potential plateaus.

2) **You're Not A Kid Anymore** – Remember those days when you were a kid and could rebound from a bike accident or broken bone in what seemed like no time at all? One of the biggest reasons for this resiliency is the amount of Human Growth Hormone (HGH) you produce as a kid. If you're over 35 years old, your body simply will not produce human growth hormone like it did when you were a kid. If this is the case, don't beat yourself up. Just make sure you address all potential diet and supplement hacks for anti-aging and take more time off to rebuild.

3) **Stress Or Illness** – If you have a lot of stress or are struggling with a virus or pathogen, chances are your body is using its resources to cope with those challenges and will not have the resources to strength train at peak performance. While most of the time this will be obvious, if you've ruled out all the other potential pitfalls of poor performance and can't seem to put your finger on the problem this could, in fact, be your challenge. If this is the case, again, you'll need to back off, take more time to rest and let your body recover.

4) **Injuries** – If you have a nagging injury or a repetitive stress injury that just doesn't want to heal, you'll need to back off and give it more time. Try waiting at least two weeks then test it out again. If this doesn't work give it another two weeks

and consider some physical therapy or massage.

If you struggle with any of the four secondary factors, make sure you adjust your recovery time. Again, don't be afraid to take 10, 14 or 21 days off before you revisit a particular exercise and muscle group.

Cold Water Therapy (AKA Cryotherapy) For Recovery

Ever noticed how professional athletes like basketball players get ice packs wrapped around their knees after every game? There's a really good reason for this, which also points us to one of the most powerful recovery and rebuilding strategies for all three disciplines of the Fired Up program.

Essentially, while localized targeted cold therapy can prevent bruising, swelling and numb pain, on a whole-body scale by immersing yourself in a cold shower, ocean, lake or bath you can bring down your heart rate, increase circulation, lower inflammation and speed up recovery. And by speeding up recovery time you can accelerate the building of more strength, which makes this one of the most prized strategies for the worlds greatest athletes.

And while you may not be a world-class athlete, if you've ever felt sore from working out or felt limited by your ability to recover, this strategy will be a game changer for expediting your superhuman powers.

Let's take a look at some of the science behind cold-water therapy and how it integrates into the Fired Up program.

The Science

You've probably experienced the uplifting effects of cold-water therapy if not directly by jumping into a cold lake, indirectly when you accidently stepped into a cold shower or a cold pool.

While this may have been shocking, according to studies, cold showers activate your sympathetic nervous system and increase the availability of neurotransmitters such as norepinephrine and endorphins, which can reverse depression and other negative emotions.[50]

As far as cold-water therapy for recovery, a landmark study analyzed 17 trials involving over 360 people who either rested or immersed themselves in cold water after resistance training, cycling or running. At the end of the study researchers concluded that cold-water baths were much more effective in relieving sore muscles one to four days after exercise than those who simply rested.[51]

And if you have a lot of stress in your life (like most of us) or suffer from getting sick often, studies also show that by exposing your whole body to cold water for short periods of time promotes "hardening," which results in increased tolerance to stress and disease.[52]

One of the most notable displays of superhuman power through cold-water therapy is Guinness Book world record holder Wim Hof who was made famous for swimming under ice, running a half-marathon barefoot on ice and being injected with a toxic virus, which had virtually no negative effect.

Interestingly enough, Wim attributes his records to a combination of frequent cold exposure, breathing techniques and meditation, which are all included as part of the Fired Up program.

And if lifting your mood, expediting recovery and making you more resistant to illness doesn't tip the scales and push you overboard, perhaps the fact that cold-water therapy has also been shown to help boost your fat-burning power will. This also includes drinking cold beverages, which force you to burn more calories as your body heats up that cold beverage (preferably without sugar).

How Cold and How Long?

Studies vary on how cold you need the water to be and how long you need to be under its influence but overall, for the bigger benefits you'll need to make it colder and stay longer.

Specifically, to acquire the bigger benefits like significant fat loss and expedited recovery you'll need to immerse yourself in water ranging in temperature from 50-65 degrees Fahrenheit (10-18 Celsius) for 15-25 minutes.

But even short bursts of cold water have been proven by studies to have a significant impact on lessening your sick days and boosting your mood.

One such study enrolled 3,018 people who took a hot shower then used applications of cold water for 30–90 seconds and found that people who take cold showers are 29% less likely to call in sick for work or school. The researchers did not find a difference between the people who took a cold shower for 30, 60, or 90 seconds. This led them to conclude that cold water triggers the body's immune system regardless of duration.[53]

With these studies in mind here's what I recommend:

1) After you workout take a warm shower just to clean off, then turn off the heat and just leave the cold on for 1-15 minutes. Since it's difficult to completely immerse your entire body make sure you isolate the water onto your upper the back of your neck as well as your upper chest for most of the time since these spots are highly conductive in lowering your overall body temperature quickly to give you maximum benefits. For a minority of the time move it around the rest of your body, especially the achy sore spots.

2) Drink ice water regularly.

3) If you have a lake or cold ocean nearby take a swim for 15-25 minutes. Check

www.MagicSeaweed.com to confirm the temperature if an ocean is nearby.

4) Try Cryotherapy from a local service. Check reviews on sites like www.Yelp.com to make sure it's legitimate and worth the price.

5) While filling a tub with cold water and ice is a more advanced strategy, if you choose this route make sure you work your way up to it. Once you do jump in, start with 10 minutes 1-2 days per week and work your way up to 3 days per week for 20-25 minutes over the next couple months.

CAUTION: If you are feeling sick, unusually weak or tired and this is unrelated to exercise or muscle fatigue, do not engage in cold-water therapy or intense strength training.

If you are feeling weak or under the weather intense strength training could compromise your immune system and throw you over the edge into a full-blown illness. If this is the case consider taking a hot bath and doing some light yoga.

As for the cold-water therapy, I learned to obey this caution the hard way when I was on vacation one summer in the Rocky Mountains of Colorado. I had been pushing my body to the limit with daily hiking, mountain biking and swimming in freezing cold water. All was good until I hit a wall of exhaustion a week later and started feeling unusually weak and tired. Instead of just taking a hot bath or shower and resting I went for a dip in the freezing cold Yampa River. While this felt great for about an hour or two after, I woke up the next day with a massive headache and had to nurse a cold for the next few days while on vacation (not so fun).

How Many Days A Week Should I Strength Train?

While we'll cover detailed recommendations for your strength training days shorty, for now, it's important to understand how you can fall prey to "Overkill" by strength training too many days of the week.

If you do not take enough time off during the week from strength training, you are putting a tremendous amount of pressure on your tendons, ligaments and muscles, which again could result in injury - perhaps even catastrophic.

While studies show the breaking down of muscle fiber as an integral part of the strength and muscle building process, these same studies also show that overtraining (Overkill) leads to reductions in speed, power, and the ability to perform exercises.[54]

Essentially, by overtraining, you're setting yourself up for failure and going backward. Again, you'll need to listen to the warning signals your body and mind provide in order to avoid this massive pitfall. To get more familiar with these signals, go ahead and take

note if you feel any of the following
symptoms:

- Trouble sleeping
- Loss of appetite and unintended
  weight loss
- Inability to focus
- Anxious, impatient, irritable or restless
- Soreness and weakness that doesn't
  go away with rest
- Irregularly slow or fast heart rate
- Depression

While these symptoms could be related to
other factors like stress or illness, studies
show that these could be from overtraining.[55]
   If this is the case, your body will let you
know. So first and foremost, listen to your
body and these warning signals, they're like
alarm clocks telling you to take better care of
yourself. Fortunately yoga will come in big in
this regard as it will help you become more
mindful and aware of potential problems
before they happen.
   Second, in addition to resting from
particular exercises and muscle groups I
recommend the following:

- **2-3 Hard Sets** – If you're doing 2-3
  hard sets, try not to exercise the same
  muscle group more than **1-2 days a
  week or less if you feel weak.**

- **1 Hard Set** – If you're doing 1 hard set
  of a particular exercise, try not to

exercise the same muscle group more than **2-4 days a week or less if you feel weak.**

This will become more clear when we get to the recommended training programs. Just know, for now, strength training with hard sets can easily lead to "Overkill," so listen to your body and allow it to fully recover before you hit those hard sets.

Do I Need To Warm-up?

While there are cases when you won't need to warm-up, when you do "hard sets" using weights, the answer is "Yes," you should warm-up.
When you first start strength training with weights, you won't be strong enough to lift a lot, which means you can probably get away with poor technique.   But once you get stronger, the increased volume of weight increases the risk of injury.
Fortunately, studies show that a short warm-up routine can significantly boost performance levels, which can translate into more muscle and strength gain over time.[56] Accordingly, to make sure each of your major muscle groups are warmed up for peak performance, in *Fired Up* you're going to do 1-2 warm-up sets prior to each hard set of a particular muscle group.
If your workout involves exercises that use the same muscle groups you will only need to warm-up on your first exercise.

For example, let's say it's a push day and you want to do bench press, overhead shoulder press and dips. And let's also say that your "hard set" weight of 4-8 reps is currently 130 pounds.

In this case, you would first warm-up for the bench press by lowering the weight to about 50% of your hard set weight (65 pounds) then slowly and with control do 10-15 reps. When you finish this first set you can do another warm-up set by adding up 80% of your "hard set" weight (100 pounds) and do one more warm-up set with 8-13 reps.

Now, you're warmed up and it's time to begin your hard sets.

Once you get to the shoulder press, you've already warmed up your press muscles with the bench press, so you can jump into your hard sets right away.

The same goes for your dips since these are also warmed up during the bench press warm-up.

When Warm-up Is Unnecessary

When you are strength training without weight you may or may not need to warm-up depending on your level of strength.

If for example, you can easily push past 8 reps of a particular exercise then you can simply apply the super slow strength training principles taught earlier and focus on proper form.

On the other hand, if you are just getting started, you can warm-up by reducing the weight of your body.

For example, push-ups can be done with your knees on the floor, pull-ups can be done with your feet on a chair and dips can be done with your feet on the floor or a chair.

In addition to giving your muscles proper time for recovery, the second most important key to avoiding injury in strength training is to make a commitment to proper form.

If you are raising and lowering the weight too quickly you are at a much higher risk for poor form and eventual injury. Make sure you watch the videos from the Fired Up program and commit to becoming a form fanatic!

Commit To Being A Form Fanatic!

What Equipment Do I Need?

At this point, we've talked about strength training routines both with and without weights. To be absolutely clear, you do not need any equipment at all to perform strength training but if it's in your budget you can amplify your gains and create more power with some very basic equipment.   Here is what I recommend:

Gym Membership – While obvious, a gym will give you access to both free-weights and machines that will allow you to do the entire *Fired Up* Strength Training program.

Multi-Use Machine – If going to the gym isn't appealing to you I understand. Personally, I don't always have the time and there a lot of distractions at the gym so occasionally I'll use my "Total Iron Gym" multifunction bar at home. This allows me to do pull-ups, chin-ups, leg raises, push-ups and dips without ever having to leave my home.

Resistance Bands – Again, if the gym isn't in the cards I recommend buying some inexpensive resistance bands, which will allow you to increase the weight and lower your reps thereby increasing both muscle and strength.

Dumbbells – For most of your strength training exercises you can use dumbbells, which I highly recommend. Even better, if you can buy ones with various weight options you can increase your options considerably. You can buy brand new multi-option dumbbells for around $50 to $500.

Bench – By giving you the support to push more weight (dumbbells or barbell) a bench will be a big asset to your workout program and you can get one for around $50.

WARNING: Don't Get Ripped Off

There is lots of low-grade cheap stuff out there so I only recommend buying from a reputable source where you can return it for no charge. I've researched the best and most affordable products and listed them on our resources page. So make sure you check them out at the link listed below before you purchase:

https://chadscottcoaching.com/resources/

CHAPTER 5 - YOGA

"A mind free from all disturbances is yoga." -
Patanjali

While yoga has somewhat recently become popular in the West, in India, it's birthplace, the practice dates back over 5,000 years and is considered by many to be one of the oldest forms of exercise and breathwork known to mankind.

Yoga actually means "union" or "connection" of mind and body. By helping you leap over the traps of triumph and advance at a much quicker pace it represents one of the most critical assets in creating superhuman powers.

For instance, should you encounter a stressful situation like a car accident, loss of job, battling a virus or family member (which could be worse), yoga can help you to become less reactive and more powerful by utilizing breath, movement and mind control.

Multiple studies have confirmed that yoga is indeed one of the most effective methods for reducing stress and anxiety and has been proven to lower levels of cortisol.[57]   And since you just learned that one of the many negative effects of stress is the need for more recovery time and the lowering of exacerbated cortisol levels, this should be even better news.

Most people know yoga as a form of exercise using a set of postures or poses (aka asana) combined with movement, but these are just two components of yoga.

In *Fired Up*, we aren't going to go into a full technical description of hundreds of yoga concepts and schools. Instead, I've condensed the most important elements into what I call "The 4 Super Powers of Yoga."

These 4 powers will help you release tension, lower stress and cortisol, build strength, mobility, energy, and testosterone while enhancing concentration, confidence, and creating new results.

The origins of these 4 elements come from the eight limbs of yoga as outlined in an ancient text called the "Yoga Sutras." If at some point in the future you develop an advanced practice, I highly recommend you explore the rest of the eight limbs.

The 4 Super Powers Of Yoga

1. Yoga postures - Asana
2. Breathwork – Pranayama
3. Self Reflection - Pratyahara
4. Concentration - Dharana

Yoga Postures - Asana

Yoga postures, or Asana, are physical positions that are either held for a period of time or linked together in a sequence of movement.

Holding or moving in and out of these postures has a host of benefits including flexibility, agility, strengthening and toning of your muscles, building bone density, improving balance, athletic performance, cardiovascular health and the prevention of injuries (amongst others).

Pranayama – Life Force

Pranayama is two concepts combined, which includes "Prana" or "Life Force" and "Yama" or "Control / Life Force Extension." While this is the literal translation, when we break it down further, "Prana" or "Life Force" is a complete study of its own, containing volumes of both scientific and spiritual studies. So in the interest of keeping it simple, we'll refer to it as "Energy."

For instance, when you go to sleep you regenerate cells, muscles, organs and wake up feeling refreshed with more energy or "Life Force," and other bonuses – like more libido. While sleeping to increase your life force is important and we'll talk about that later, you can manipulate oxygen by channeling it with various yogic breathing techniques (AKA breathwork) to increase your energy at any time.

Pranayama is all about gaining mastery over your breath, which essentially means recognizing the connection between your breath, your mind, your body and your emotions.

For example, notice what happens with your breath when you're stressed, fearful or contemplating a difficult task that is unfamiliar. Your heart will most likely beat more rapidly, your muscles will tense up and your breath will become shorter because you're probably nervous and guess what happens when you're nervous?

Most of your oxygen is redirected to your extremities preparing you for fight or flight while your brain gets the short end of the oxygen stick, which makes it more difficult to think clearly. Regrettably, when you can't think clearly you make poor decisions or no decisions and more often than not, get regrettable results.

To avoid this pitfall, in *Fired Up,* we'll be doing breathwork with an ancient breathing technique called Ujjayi Breathing, which is one of the quickest ways to lower stress, become confident and make better decisions.

Pratyahara - Self Reflection

If you live in a developed country, chances are you've been exposed to and conditioned by multiple influences from your external world. This could range from what your friends and family think of you, to the media and advertisers who tell you how your life should or shouldn't be, which is all coming from outside of you.

Sadly, most of what your external influences believe is not serving you.

For example, for every "yes you're awesome" you more than likely get four of: "you're not that great," or "you're broken," or "you're not smart enough, tall enough, rich enough or beautiful enough, etc."

Fortunately, with self-reflection, you can toss all that garbage from the outside world into the proverbial waste can and celebrate since Pratyahara gives you more superpowers.

Self-reflection or Pratyahara simply means go within. This practice allows you to let go of all the delusions and false limiting beliefs that you should somehow be perfect or fully enlightened. And instead of constantly looking outside for approval or domination, you can look within at yourself and ask: am I present and engaged 100% in what I'm doing right now or am I worried about the past or the future or what everyone thinks of me?

Other not so obvious questions during self-reflection may also arise such as:

- Am I progressing in life?
- Am I conducting myself like a good human being?
- Am I really happy with my work?
- Am I really happy with my relationships?
- What area of life am I holding back in and how can I advance to become truly happy and successful?

With a good teacher, yoga can help you self reflect and let go of all the BS and clutter that drags you down in life and instead, really step up and savor each moment of life.

Dharana - Concentration

When in space, astronauts engage in hours upon hours of "Earth gazing."
As you can imagine, looking at the earth from afar is most likely quite captivating, mesmerizing, perhaps even a spiritual experience (especially if you see an alien).

According to a 2018 paper called "The Overview Effect Awe and Self Transcendent Experience in Space Flight," astronauts return to Earth with a new perspective and sense of purpose from all that earth gazing.

Regrettably, when we gaze upon the common earthling here on planet Earth we find a large percentage of the population mesmerized by their smartphones, engaged in social media or some other form of entertainment, which doesn't serve them. And instead of building concentration, taking bold action and making dreams a reality, we may find ourselves on the couch with ADD (attention deficit disorder) looking for the next distraction (sweets, drugs, liquor) with no semblance of action or purpose.

However, in order to get *Fired Up*, make more money, find love or achieve any type of success we must concentrate for extended periods of time.

This, of course, brings us to Dharana or yogic concentration, which similar to Earth gazing, can evoke a higher state of consciousness and give you more superpowers.

Specifically, concentration is acquired when you engage in all three of the prior components (postures, breathwork and self-reflection) and begin to let go of all the distractions from past and future and fuse with the present.

For example, when doing Lord of the Dance Pose (Natarajasana), you will need to stand on one leg while holding your other leg with one hand. You'll also need to focus on your breath in order to calm your mind and let go of distractions. Finally, you'll need to concentrate your eyes on one point for and extended period of time.

As a natural consequence of this mental and physical challenge, you'll begin to self-reflect and notice when your mind wants to freak out because the strain is too challenging or you lose your balance.

Over time, as you practice yoga, you'll become aware of your negative tendencies like overreacting, breathing shallow, looking all over the place and comparing yourself to others. This practice will eventually help you to correct your mistakes and become more calm, collected, clear-headed, decisive, centered, focused, present and most importantly… confidant!

So let's say in the past your tendency was pushing yourself too hard (Overkill) just because someone else in the class was more advanced than you. But once you incorporate the 4 Super Powers of Yoga, your new level of self-reflection and concentration begin to help you gauge just the right amount of push to challenge you and create growth, while at the same time, protecting you from injury.

Or let's say your tendency wasn't overkill, instead, you just did whatever you felt was within your comfort zone.

Once you practice yoga regularly (from a good teacher), you'll start to interrupt long standing mental patterns of freaking out from fear. You'll also have the added skill of breathwork to master your mind and its emotions, which will help you avoid the ravaging effects of cortisol and stress. At this point, you'll more than likely take a leap forward, try something new and experience the true joy of following your passions and freely expressing yourself (not to mention all the success that comes with that).

The Awesomeness

We already mentioned how the combined synergistic effects of the 4 Super Powers of Yoga can radically alter your health for the better by reducing tension and stress but there are other superpowers you should know about. Make sure you don't just read these but instead, imagine them in your life. By doing this you'll have a much better chance at committing to a regular practice.

Counteracts Flexion Dominance, Low Self-Esteem & Low Energy

Flexion is the position you find yourself in throughout the day when you're driving, texting, cooking, watching TV or hunched over a keyboard.

As you can imagine, leaning forward for long periods of time eventually takes a toll on your joints and muscles but you may be surprised to learn that it can lead to depression, low self-esteem and low energy. If you're at all doubtful about how important good posture is perhaps the following studies will convince you otherwise.

Turns out, over 55 published studies prove poor posture has negative consequences and open expansive posture created from a regular yoga practice leads to multiple benefits. Below are five of my favorites; as you read through them, notice which ones relate to your personal circumstances.

- **Self-Esteem Study** – Researchers stated in a 2015 stud published by Health Psychology: "Slouchers reported significantly lower self-esteem, mood, and greater fear."

- **Confidence Study -** A 2012 study by scientists Pablo Binol, Richard Petty, and Benjamin Wagner on how body posture might affect "self-evaluation" showed that people who stood in a power pose (they called it "confident posture," with chest pushed out and erect spine) were much more prone to rate themselves more confidently than people in a "doubtful posture," slumped and self-contained.

- **Low Energy & Body Pain Study -** Published in Biofeedback in 2017 by Dr. Erik Peper, this study found that "Sitting up straight" led to "positive thoughts and memories" while a sad, slumped walk "decreased energy levels." The study also found that poor posture could lead to fatigue, headaches, poor concentration, increased muscle tension and over time injury to your vertebrae.

- **Power Study -** When scientists tried to poke holes in Harvard University professor Amy Cuddy's study from 2012 proving good posture makes you more powerful she created a follow-up study published by Sage Journals Psychological Science in 2017. This study examined over 55 additional studies and clearly demonstrates: "A link between expansive, open postures and feelings of power."

- **Depression Study -** A study published by the Journal of Behavior Therapy and Experimental Psychiatry in 2017 found that: "Adopting an upright posture may increase positive affects, reduce fatigue, and decrease self-focus in people with mild-to-moderate depression"

Fortunately, one of the main highlights of yoga and the *Fired Up* program is its many postures, which counteract this flexion dominance and boost your mood, energy and confidence.

Lowers Cortisol and Stress

Further study conducted by Russian scientists in 2001 examined the effects of the Cobra pose on the hormone levels of healthy subjects. In the experiment, researchers drew blood from a group of seven volunteers both before and after they did the Cobra pose. In their report, they determined that cortisol levels dropped in the volunteers by an average of 11% after holding the pose for just 2-3 minutes.

Increases Testosterone

Perhaps even more interesting was the fact that researchers in the same study found the subjects testosterone levels increased by an average of 16%, with one male subject experiencing a 33% increase and the lone female in the study experiencing a whopping 55% increase. This is obviously significant as increasing testosterone helps increase libido and lowering cortisol reduces your stress levels. But it gets even better.

Reduces Fear & Regulates Emotions

Several studies show that yoga effects and changes parts of your brain, which most other forms of exercise, simply do not.

For example, one study reviewed over two decades of research and found that yoga postures (asana) and breathwork (pranayama) reduced amygdala volume on the right hand side of the brain, which is associated with negative emotions and fear. [58]

Another study from Stanford University showed similar results of a reduction in fear through concentration and self-reflection (Dharana and Pratyahara) by being more mindful of emotions instead of simply burying them or running from them. [59]

Essentially, by engaging in a mindful yoga practice like the ones in the Fired Up Program you'll activate all four superpowers of yoga and reduce fear, which holds you back from success and really experiencing life at the peak.

Increases Confidence

To further bolster the fear reduction claim, it's worth mentioning important research from Harvard University, The University of Oregon and The University of Texas which concluded that powerful and effective leaders (men and women) not only share similar mindsets, but also similar hormone levels.

More specifically, researchers discovered that: "Powerful leaders tend to have higher levels of testosterone, which leads to more confidence, and lower levels of cortisol, which leads to better coping skills for high stress situations." [60] [61] And since we know all three elements of *Fired Up* boost testosterone you can count on a healthy dose of confidence flowing through your veins after your daily practice.

Once you develop a regular yoga practice, the real benefit is that it not only feels really good all over but it translates into more confidence when speaking in front of people, trying something new, getting up on stage, taking on a leadership role, calling someone out for being dishonest or overcoming any other life challenge. After teaching well over 10,000 students I can personally attest to this as a common occurrence.

Relieves Back Pain

Chances are if you've been to your doctor for a back problem, they did not recommend dead lifts or HIIT to fix your problem. Instead, they more than likely recommended yoga. This is because, unlike other forms of exercise, yoga has been proven through multiple studies to relieve chronic back pain.[62] Considering the fact that back pain is one of the most common disabling injuries and is a leading cause of lost productivity, this should be really good news.

Makes You Feel Really Good

While yoga produces feel good chemicals like endorphins, by adding in The 4 Super Powers of Yoga, when you engage in the *Fired Up* classes you will feel a different high than you will from Strength Training and HIIT.

Almost without exception, I find most of my students report that they simply can't get that high from strength training or HIIT. Hopefully, this piques your interest and gets you even further committed.

Better Friends and Influences

A perhaps less tangible but clearly measurable benefit is the new friends and influences from the yoga community who lift you up instead of drag you down.

Remember, whoever you surround yourself with has a direct impact on your results or lack thereof. So once you start to get comfortable with the videos provided in this training, I suggest you go to an actual class and experience the energy of other people doing the same thing you're doing. This will fulfill an additional need we all have for "love and connection" - more superpower!

Keep in mind, your first experience may not be so great simply because some teachers are just getting started and some are just not your style or pace. Some teachers get bogged down in talking about things that may not appeal to you, yet some are really experienced and speak just enough without distracting you from concentrating. You'll need to keep searching and taking classes with different teachers until you find one that resonates with you.

Hopefully after taking the Fired Up classes you'll understand what a good teacher actually does, which will give you something to measure other teachers against.

Yoga Is The Glue Of Life

We also mentioned the physical benefits of postures like flexibility, agility, strength, balance and cardiovascular health but even more important is the synergy created when these effects are combined.

Effectively, when you practice yoga regularly, it insulates and protects you from injury, illness and disease while making everything else in life easier including the other two disciplines of *Fired Up* – Strength Training and HIIT.

If we simply look to the highest level of performance in society like professional sports, we see athletes in the NFL, NBA, MBL, ATP and NHL who have embraced yoga as regular practice simply because it gives you a distinct advantage both on and off the field.

Eventually, as you progress in your own practice you too will come to see how yoga can be the glue of your life!

Yoga For Life - Bullet Proofing Beliefs

"In truth, yoga doesn't take time, it gives time"
– Ganga White

Whether you add time to your life and make everything easier with a regular yoga practice or waste your life away on the couch depends in large part on your beliefs. So again, it's time to look at your underlying beliefs and make absolutely sure nothing stands in the way of you and your superpowers.

Time For Action

Below are the four critical questions you'll need to answer in order to start the belief change process. If you're at all unsure about how to answer a question just reference the examples provided.

1) How did your old belief play out in a Circle of Results Model?

When it comes to limiting beliefs about yoga, there is quite a bit of stigma and misguided information. To ensure you don't fall into any of these traps I'm going to list some limiting beliefs below. Make sure you are absolutely honest if you've ever felt or experienced these beliefs.

I'm Not Flexible, I Can't Do Yoga - Have you ever heard someone, perhaps even yourself say something like, "I'm not flexible I can't do yoga?" This is like saying: "I'm not hydrated because I can't drink water."

People are not inflexible because they're just born that way. In reality, babies and children are extremely flexible. The only reason people are inflexible is simply because they do not stretch or do yoga.

Complicating the problem is the fact that the longer you wait, the more inflexible you become and the more inflexible you become the less likely you are to start a yoga practice.

The simple fact is, if you do not stretch your muscles, over time you will find yourself in some real pain that might not be reversible.

For example, my friends Dad led a sedentary life for a long time. He, like most of us, spent a lot of time hunched over while driving, sitting, painting, watching TV and using a computer. Eventually, without ever using counter postures like "Cobra" his spine fused together in a hunched position. So remember this one:

The more inflexible you are, the more you need yoga!

Yoga Is Just For Ladies - Another misguided belief is that yoga is just for ladies. And while yoga's primary practitioners in countries like the United States and Canada may indeed be women, in India, its birthplace, the primary practitioners are actually men.

Furthermore, if we simply retrace yoga's history we find pioneers like Patanjali,

Pattabhi Jois and BKS Iyengar who were all men. The only real reason men are just starting to catch on to the incredible benefits of yoga is because of stigma.

In other words, most men fall prey to the illusion that if women do it, it's probably too feminine and therefore it can't be good for men. In reality, nothing could be further from the truth.

I've been teaching yoga for over 13 years and I'm still blown away by how few guys have caught onto the power of yoga. There's a good reason why it's practiced by media moguls like Russell Simons and Richard Branson, athletes like LeBron James and Ray Lewis, musicians like Sting and Adam Levine, actors like Robert Downey Jr. and Jennifer Aniston, world leaders and people like you and me. Because it works!

Yoga Is Religious - Yoga has many branches, disciplines, and founders, yet there are no mandatory rules on how to practice it. Through its evolution, people have added dimensions and branches to expand the experience of yoga beyond just physical postures and movements. As mentioned earlier in The 4 Super Powers of Yoga, this includes Patanjali who lived in India around 400 CE (roughly 200 AD) and synthesized knowledge about yoga from older traditions into what is now called the 8-limbs or "Yoga Sutras."

In *Fired Up* we'll be using four of the most crucial components from the yoga canon, which do not have any religious affiliation, yet will allow you to develop strength, mobility, concentration and unbreakable confidence.

Yoga Is Boring Or Too Easy - You may have watched or been personally involved in a yoga class that looked like you could take a nap and still do the class. And while some classes like restorative are indeed very slow, we'll be focusing on a wide range of classes for different purposes, whether that be restoring energy, healing, strengthening, balancing or getting fired up.

For example, you may have had a long day at work and instead of heading straight to the couch and fusing your spine into the hunchback position, you choose a 45-minute energizer class, which fires you up to then go work on your passions instead of wasting your life watching someone else live theirs.

Circle of Results Model Example

Below is an example of a Circle of Results Model, which answers question #1 using an example from above. As you read it, take a note on how you can use this format to craft your own model.

1) What did you pretend to believe which when realized would make this disempowered belief go away forever?

B - I pretended to believe that Yoga was just for women and feminine men. I pretended to believe that I wasn't limber so I couldn't do it. In reality, deep down I knew that the only reason I wasn't limber was because I wasn't willing to do yoga. I also used to believe it was like a cultish religion so I avoided it.

T – I thought, if I do yoga I'll be looked at like I'm a wimp and I'll just embarrass myself.

E – I feel anxious and doubtful

A – I stay away from yoga and talk about it like it's for ladies and wussies

R – I remain inflexible with a lot of pain in my lower back. I'm judgmental and don't try new things, which puts me on the couch with a lot of depression and helplessness.

Write down your "Old Belief" in a Circle of Results Model.

____

2) What are the problems created by your old belief?

Describe the problems your old belief created – i.e., how much time was wasted, any bad habits you developed, how did you suffer, how did it make you feel?

For example: I used to waste countless hours on the couch binge watching sports and overeating pizza. I must have wasted 10 hours a week for 8 years, which could've been spent working on my dreams and building my dream business – a bike shop with specialty cruisers. I also gained a lot of weight and neglected to stretch, which limited my mobility and threw my back out regularly. I felt stuck so I didn't take much new action.

Write Down The Problems Created by Your Old Belief

____

3) What are the benefits of your problem?

If there were a benefit to having this problem what would it be? Is there something that your unconscious mind wants you to understand that if you understood it would make the problem disappear?

For example: I realized that I was just scared of being judged and that I'd lose my friends. I realized I was playing a small game by not stepping up and taking care of myself. I realized that if I was ever going to feel really good about myself and live without regrets I needed to ditch some of the bad influences in my life. I came to understand that people who criticized others for doing yoga were really just insecure about themselves. I learned that failure from the past doesn't mean failure in the future. This new perspective allowed me to step my game up, take action and start building myself with *The Power Diet* and the *Fired Up* program.

Write Down The Benefits Of Your Problem

____

____

New Belief Change Declaration #1 – Yoga Is The Glue Of Life

Now its time to declare your new belief by writing it down in a Circle of Results Model and then focus on it daily.

4) How will your "New Belief" play out in a Circle of Results Model?

Example:

B – I believe the fear of embarrassment and rejection is just a story, an excuse to remain stuck. I also believe in myself without the need for approval from others. I believe yoga is essential for men and women to maintain spinal integrity get rid of stress and lower cortisol. I believe it makes me calm, less reactive and more confident. I believe without yoga my body starts to seize up and I start to age rapidly. I also believe yoga helps me meet interesting people who inspire me to expand and grow into my full potential... it is the glue of life.

T – I think if someone judges me, it's really just a sign of insecurity. I think about how I can't wait to stretch my stiff body, feel alive and pain free.

E – I feel excited like I really found a solution I can always count on to feel good no matter what the situation.

A – I read the *Fired Up Manual* and start doing the yoga video training.

R – Within 30 days of starting the *Fired Up* program I start to see noticeable changes in my mind and body. I feel calmer, more relaxed and confident. People start to ask: "What's different about you?" They respect me more and want what I have. This gives me more confidence to take more action and pursue my passions. The extra energy and confidence gives me the courage to start that bike shop I've always wanted and I feel unstoppable.

Now write down a Circle of Results Model using your "New Belief":

New Belief: What do you declare as your new belief? Make sure you use Pain, Pleasure and Purpose as well as the Master

Mindsets that feel most empowering to you.

____

Thought: Describe the thoughts you'll have after you've embedded this new belief.

____
____

Emotion: Describe how you will feel once this new belief is part of your permanent mindset.

____

Action: What have you been unwilling to do in order to keep this problem? Describe the action you will take which will lead to a new habit.

____
____

Result: How do you know for sure that your old belief is no longer a problem for you? Visualize your new outcome in detail – i.e., where will you be, who will be with you, any new habits created from the action, how will you feel?

Take Action

Congratulations you've just created a new empowered belief about yoga.

I mentioned this earlier in our first belief change but since repetition is the mother of all skill, I'll repeat it again.

In order to embed this belief deep into your subconscious and make it a more permanent part of your roots, you'll need to repeat it to yourself daily for 90 days, which will create a long-term habit.

What I recommend is you write your Circle of Results Model down in your smartphone on a notepad.

Next, open your electronic calendar and write a reminder that repeats every day for the next 90 days. All you have to do is read the note when that reminder pops up, it's really that simple.

To make it even more effective, try to memorize it and repeat it out loud to yourself.

Last but definitely not least, make absolutely sure you tell a friend or family member about your new belief and how you are committed to keeping it. This is absolutely crucial as studies show telling others about a goal helps you stay accountable and committed to upholding that belief.

Take action on this and do not hesitate. Make the call!

Simple Breathwork Using Ujjayi Breathing Technique

Hopefully, at this point, you're Fired Up and ready to jump into a yoga class. But before you do it's important to set yourself up for success.

Since breathwork is such an integral part of yoga and the *Fired Up* program, we're going to take moment right now to practice Ujjayi breathing. Again, this will make everything easier, including your yoga practice so don't skip out here.

If it's any consolation, after teaching over 10,000 yoga students, I can say with 100% certainty that the people who struggle the most are the ones who do not know how to breathe properly.

How it works

Ujjayi Breathing stimulates your PNS or parasympathetic nervous system, which as we mentioned earlier, is responsible for processes like rest, digest and rejuvenation.

In contrast, your SNS or sympathetic nervous system is what kicks in high gear when you are fearful, threatened or become stressed out. This is the fight or flight part of your nervous system, which siphons blood from your core and moves it into your limbs so you can either fight or run away from a threat.

Considering the demands of today's hustle and bustle challenges like road rage, job dissatisfaction, relationship stress and poor health topped off with the constant distraction of social media, we are currently experiencing an SNS crisis with very little to show for in the PNS department.

Fortunately, Ujjayi breathing addresses this dilemma head on by pulling oxygen deep into the lower lobes of your lungs where the PNS is highly concentrated. And while the *Fired Up* program will give instruction on synchronizing this process with yoga postures, you can do Ujjayi breathing alone when stressed, anxious, experiencing insomnia or as part of a daily practice.

Of course, that's not all Ujjayi is good for; it also works wonders for sexual stamina and delaying your orgasms. There's a good reason why PNS sounds like penis – It helps your penis delay ejaculation (if you have one)!

I found this out purely out of experimentation when I was having sex with my girlfriend one day.

I was overly excited and just started breathing really deeply using the Ujjayi Breathing technique. Shortly thereafter, like magic, everything calmed down, I was able to enjoy sex much longer, with more stamina and confidence.

When you think about it, this actually makes sense. When you use Ujjayi Breathing technique you are stimulating your PNS and relaxing your muscles, including everything associated with intercourse and ejaculation. This one little trick made a huge difference in my sexual performance and won me huge points with my gal so take this one seriously and practice it to perfection.

And for all the ladies out there, make sure you share this tip with your man; you'll be glad you did!

To get started I suggest watching the video on Ujjayi breathing in the *Fired Up* program but I will also describe the step-by-step process here for further clarification.

1) Get Set Up - Go ahead and turn your phone on silent then find a place where you won't be bothered. Try not to wear restrictive or tight clothes as this can hinder your progress. Either sit in a chair or in a cross-legged position on a pillow or blanket, preferably with your hips above your knees for good blood circulation, otherwise, you may get uncomfortable quickly.

2) Test The Rise & Fall Of Your Diaphragm - As a professional singer for over 20 years and having been trained by one of the best vocal coaches in the world, I learned that to sustain your breath you need to breathe from your diaphragm rather than your chest or throat.

To test this, go ahead and close your eyes then place your hands one on top of the other on your navel so you can feel the expansion of your diaphragm when you breathe. Now inhale into your diaphragm and notice if you feel your belly rise. Keep trying until it's clear you are breathing from your diaphragm rather than your chest or throat.

Once you verify it's working you can extend your arms in front palms up or down as a gesture of receiving or grounding. In yoga, these are called "Mudras" and symbolize your intention to find grounding (palms down) when you're feeling anxious or stressed or receive something (palms up) like better health, more wealth or loving relationships.

3) Create Oceanic Resonance – Next, we're going to work on creating some resonance when you inhale and exhale. This is the most important part of the breathwork so pay close attention here. To achieve this, when you breathe, think about creating a slight snoring sound on your inhale by constricting (slightly closing) the back of your throat. This isn't a full snore, just enough to create a slight resonance.

Next, on your exhale try to say "HA" like you're opening your mouth for the dentist, without actually opening your mouth. You should hear a distinct sound or resonance. Now let's begin the cycle of breath.

Go ahead and breathe in through your nose with your mouth closed and direct this breath into your abdomen or lower belly while constricting the back of your throat and lifting your tongue to the roof of your mouth. If your hand is on your belly you should feel it rise upward.

Let the oxygen expand your abdomen then gradually fill up your lungs, chest, and throat. To exhale, again you're going to keep your mouth closed and try to make the "Ha" sound while allowing the oxygen to slowly release through your nose.

Once you start to feel the rise and fall of your diaphragm and belly and you hear a slight resonance from constricting the back of your throat on your inhale and exhale you're on the right path so keep going.

4) Lengthen Your Breath - Next, it's time to focus on lengthening your breath and make both your inhale and exhale last longer. This, of course, translates directly into the activation of your PNS, which relaxes your body and mind, allows for better decision making and creates a calm and confident state of mind.

To do this, first, just count the seconds it takes to inhale and exhale. Your inhale will always be a bit shorter than your exhale so try to inhale for a minimum of 4 counts but shoot to eventually increase this to 10 or more counts.

On your exhale try for a minimum of 5 counts then shoot for 12 or more counts as you advance. Once you have a good long breath go ahead and drop the counting and use some guided imagery of the ocean tide coming in with your inhale and going out with your exhale. At this point you should have only two things to focus on:

1. The sound (resonance) of your breath
2. The image (ocean tide) of your breath

If your mind wanders, and it most likely will, just remember that there is a process to improvement. Just like anything else you learn that is new and different, real change takes time and effort. Breathwork is no different. You will get better at it, but only if you do it consistently.

If you've read my book <u>Get High On Confidence</u>, you'll remember a concept called "Deliberate Practice," which simply means practice what you're not good at until you're good at it. While deliberate practice is key in forming a new habit and developing superpowers, without the right beliefs, you'll most likely get sidetracked by those Traps of Triumph. As such, it's now time to shore up any holes in your belief system so your lifeboat doesn't capsize on the way to your island full of treasure.

Once you have a good idea of how to breathe using the Ujjayi technique you can refer to the video training in the Fired Up program, which will show you how to integrate The 4 Super Powers of Yoga.

How Often Should I Practice Yoga?

As far as frequency is concerned, unlike HIIT and Strength Training, you can do yoga every day.

For example, let's say you are taking Sunday off to rest and recover. This doesn't mean you just sit on the couch for 12 hours and watch football or figure skating. In fact, if you do this your hamstrings will be extremely tight and set you up for a back injury. In addition, normal blood flow and your body's ability to detoxify will slow down and similar to a swamp that attracts mosquitoes, you're body will be a prime palace to attract lots of disease and distress.

In this case, you could simply follow one of the restorative classes or do a quick 30-minute class from the *Fired Up* program library.

Can You Stretch Too Much?

Yes, just like anything in life, if you do it too much you can create a negative effect. In Yoga, this is called "Hypermobility," which several studies have linked to chronic pain.[63] [64] As such, there are two main instances you should avoid both of which fall into the "Overkill" trap.

Overstretching Once – When it comes to flexibility and stretching, the goal of yoga is to stretch muscles and fascia not tendons, joints or ligaments. Unsurprisingly, overstretching occurs when you push past the elasticity limits of muscles, joints and ligaments, which can then lead to an injury.

For example, I've witnessed dozens of students come to my class and attempt pigeon pose but simply aren't ready for it. This is a deep knee bend that opens your hips and if you allow your ego to take over when you're not quite ready, you may find yourself with overstretched ligaments and tendons that do not recover.

If you feel a sharp pain or numbness, back off and go easy. This means you are stretching joints and ligaments as opposed to the middle of the muscle.   In the *Fired Up* program, I will give you alternatives, which take into consideration ability level and potential injuries.

So for example, in the case of pigeon pose, I would recommend reverse pigeon, which is performed on your back without the added pressure of your body on top of your knee.

Overstretching with Frequency – The second potential pitfall of "Overkill" occurs when you do the same thing (no matter how safe) too many times in too short a time period.

Similar to repetitive stress injuries, if you do up dog 50 times a day 7 days a week, no matter how good it is for you, you may find that the pressure on your wrists starts to negatively affect the surrounding ligaments and tendons. Make sure you pay special attention to the workout recommendations at the end of this manual so you don't fall prey to overkill.

Equipment

Again, you don't need to buy anything if it's not in the budget. You can do yoga on a towel, carpet, wood, cement or grass. That being said, yoga is going to be your new secret weapon and there is only 1 key piece of equipment you absolutely need – a yoga mat.

I suggest you invest about $60 in a good yoga mat, which will protect your knees and give your feet good grip. If you buy a good one from our resources page it should last a lifetime.

Additionally, I recommend buying a couple of foam blocks, especially for beginner to intermediate practitioners. This will allow you to perform postures that would be impossible for most and save you from unnecessary injuries. To check out my best recommendations visit:
www.chadscottcoaching.com/resources

CHAPTER 6 – HIGH INTENSITY INTERVAL TRAINING (HIIT)

"Inspiration is a guest that does not willingly visit the lazy."
— Tchaikovsky

Of the three disciplines that comprise the *Fired Up* program, High intensity interval training (HIIT) could be the most misunderstood and misguided of them all. Unfortunately, poor instruction and high impact variations have led to a lot of injuries, which in turn has contributed to a lot of fear and avoidance.

Fortunately, HIIT is a well-documented strategy for improving health, building lean muscle, burning fat and increasing endurance. [65] And by following the *Fired Up* protocol you can avoid the injuries and gain its amazing benefits.

How does it work?

HIIT's almost magical ability to boost your superpowers comes from the alternation of short work intervals, which push your heart rate up to 70-90% of its maximum and longer recovery periods that slow your heart rate down to 60-70% of its maximum. By rotating these intervals, HIIT allows you to workout for less time than traditional methods like jogging, aerobics and many other forms of exercise while achieving superior results.

The Awesomeness

There's a good reason why HIIT has become so popular. It's got some solid studies and unique effects, which can multiply your superpowers.   As you read the benefits below, similar to Yoga and Strength Training, don't just read them; instead, imagine yourself with these benefits and how they would affect your life.

Utilizes Both Anaerobic and Aerobic Systems

HIIT is considered to be much more effective than normal cardio because it alternates the activation of your aerobic and anaerobic endurance systems and multiplies the benefits. This is highly significant since you don't have to tax your body by running 10 miles every day to get the benefits of cardiovascular health.

Boosts Your Immunity and Increases Heart Health

Nitric oxide is produced by just about every type of cell in your body and acts as a vasodilator, which means it causes your blood vessels to expand and dilate. This, in turn, increases blood flow and lowers your blood pressure, which makes it one of the most important molecules for blood vessel health.

Of course, HIIT increases nitric oxide production as published in several studies including one with 16 young sedentary males in 2013, which found that six weeks of HIIT led to a 36% increase in endothelial nitric oxide synthase (eNOS) while Endurance Training over the same time period only led to a 16% increase.[66]

One of the greatest benefits of nitric oxide is that it boosts immune function and helps you fight off invaders like the Coronavirus. And since heart disease is the #1 cause of death you may find yourself doubling down on HIIT since the nitric oxide it creates stimulates the thinning of your blood and decreases blood viscosity, which in turn decreases platelet aggregation (a good thing)!

Boosts Erections

If you've read my book "Man Up – The Ultimate Guide To Natural ED Cures," you'll have learned that men must absolutely must have good blood flow in order to have an erection, not to mention reduce the risk of a life-threatening blood clot, which means HIIT could be you and your significant other's new best friend.

Burns Excess Fat

Nitric oxide is also a primary contributor to fat loss due to its powerful anabolic stimulus, which is known to help increase your lean body mass. Additionally, increased muscle mass helps your body burn fat for fuel.

In research studies, HIIT has been shown to burn adipose tissue more effectively than low-intensity exercise (up to 50% more efficiently). Additionally, it has been shown to speed up your metabolism, which helps you burn more calories throughout the day.

Another interesting study from Laval University in Quebec, Canada found that "HIIT cardio helped trainees lose nine times more fat than those who trained the traditional way with moderate speed for 20-60 minutes."

Slows Down Aging

If losing nine times more weight than traditional cardio doesn't get you excited maybe turning back the aging clock will.

According to Dr. Joe Mercola "Nitric oxide may also assist with counteracting mitochondrial decline because exercise forces your mitochondria to replicate themselves in response to the higher energy requirement demanded by the workout. Even though aging is inevitable, the ability exercise has to spur positive mitochondrial changes may help slow some of the effects of biological aging."

Additionally, Mercola says: "Because exercise can promote mitochondrial biogenesis in the brain, it has been shown to positively contribute to the reduction or reversal of age-associated decline in cognitive function and assist in repairing brain damage after a stroke."

Increases HGH

We talked about HGH earlier in Strength Training as a superhero of hormones and by adding yet another trigger for HGH you'll start to see how the synergy of these three disciplines starts to really work in your favor.

Specifically, by boosting HGH with all three of the disciplines in *Fired Up* you will have the combined effect of all three, which is much greater than any one individually. And when it comes to boosting HGH with HIIT there are several studies to support its production including a study from Brunel University, which showed how exercise "training above the lactate threshold may amplify the pulsatile release of HGH at rest, increasing 24-hour HGH secretion".[67]

In other words, short bouts of intense training (HIIT) can increase HGH after the exercise and for up to 24 hours.

Another revealing study from Loughborough University compared the effect of a single 6 second and 30 second sprint on a stationary exercise bike and found a remarkable 450% increase in HGH after the 30 second sprint over the 6 second sprint.[68]

And if you're intimidated by sprints, don't worry, you won't need to do any. Because of their abrasive nature and notorious reputation for injury, I simply do not recommend them. In the long run, you're better off saving your knees and avoiding a future knee replacement by using the low impact versions offered in the *Fired Up* program.

Increases Your Stamina

If you're feeling old or tired, like you just can't last that long, HIIT increases stamina and endurance by increasing your VO2 max. This is the maximum amount of oxygen your body can handle while exercising. Kind of important, when you're trying to achieve something important in life (like your dreams).

Reduces Insulin Resistance and Potential for Diabetes

Several studies show that the fat burning power of HIIT helps decrease insulin resistance, a known precursor to Type 2 diabetes. I don't know about you but the thought of drawing blood with a needle for the rest of my life to manage diabetes just doesn't sound so inviting. And if you already have diabetes, several studies show that exercise can manage it and potentially reverse it completely.[69]

Helps Athletes

Studies show HIIT "improves athletic performance by improving muscle power."[70] And while all three disciplines from *Fired Up* will help all athletes gain a competitive advantage, HIIT is specifically beneficial for athletes who play sports where the intensity varies constantly, like basketball, baseball, soccer, skiing, tennis and hockey. In this case, athletes can expect to perform better in their given sport and will typically outperform others toward the end of games when everyone else is getting tired and hitting the skids.

HIIT For Life – Bullet Proofing Beliefs

"Intensity builds immensity" – Kevin Levrone

When I first introduce my clients to the *Fired Up* program, typically their lives are not where they want them to be. But without exception, by adding the right amount of intensity, they are all pleasantly surprised at how immensely their lives begin to change for the better. This includes their relationships, their finances and their vitality to live life at a much higher vibration. This will become absolutely clear to you as well once you commit to a regular HIIT practice.

So again, before we jump into the workouts, it's absolutely crucial you address any potential traps of triumph here by creating bulletproof beliefs that insulate you from laziness, depression or the call of the couch and that bag of chips.

Time For Action

Below are the four critical questions you'll need to answer in order to start the belief change process. If you're at all unsure about how to answer a question just reference the examples provided.

1) How did your old belief play out in a Circle of Results Model?

Similar to yoga, when it comes to limiting beliefs about HIIT, there is quite a bit of stigma and misguided information circulated in the media. To ensure you don't fall into any of these traps I'm going to list some limiting beliefs below. Make sure you are absolutely honest if you've ever felt or experienced any of these.

It's Too Intense and Makes You Barf

Perhaps you've seen F45 or P90x commercials or people doing HIIT on YouTube and thought, this stuff is just too intense, too extreme and you know what? You're right!

Most of these programs fall into the "Overkill" trap and set you up for energy depletion and injury demotion. This is because HIIT only returns maximum benefits within a short period of time.

Remember the wound example from Strength Training? If you just keep pushing at maximum intensity past the maximum return on investment time, you're actually going backward and creating a wound that may never heal or just create a serious injury.

So instead of doing 40-60 minutes or more of HIIT and pushing yourself to barf, in Fired Up we only do what is necessary for maximum benefits.

It Creates Injuries

Sitting on the sidelines is certainly no fun. Unfortunately, more often than not, "Overkill" creates injuries! But the reason doesn't just come from doing something too long; it also comes from the degree of impact that the exercise delivers to your joints, muscles and bones.

For example, sprinting or doing box jumps may function as explosive plyometric exercises but the high impact they produce creates a much higher degree of risk for injury, especially if you're over 40 years old.

For this reason, *Fired Up* offers several different levels of impact from low to mid to high, so anyone can do it.

I'm Too Old

Again, as you just learned, with low impact short HIIT routines, anyone can do it, including my 75-year-old father. That's right, 75 years old. And if he can do it so can you. If you don't believe it, you may just be stuck with a limiting belief from all the misinformation circulating in the media, which we'll shortly dispose of.

I Don't Have The Energy

The problem with this belief is similar to believing you can't do yoga because you're not flexible. Barring any issues of illness, poor diet, lack of sleep or over exercising, if you're low on energy it's more than likely because you don't exercise enough.

It's Just For Athletes

By this time it should be pretty clear that with the variety of options offered by Fired Up, anyone can do HIIT. And the fact that it burns more fat in a shorter period of time than any other form of exercise should cast any remaining doubts aside and help you make a lifetime commitment.

Circle of Results Model Example

Below is an example of a Circle of Results Model, which answers question #1 using an example from above. As you read it, take a note on how you can use this format to craft your own model.

2 **What did you pretend to believe which when realized would make this disempowered belief go away forever?**

B – I pretended to believe that HIIT was just for athletes and young people who could sprint and jump until they felt nauseous.

T – I thought, if I do HIIT I'm going to feel sick and sore for a very long time and I'll just embarrass myself.

E – I feel anxious and doubtful

A – I stay away from HIIT and talk about it like it's for extreme people.

R – I remain slow, lethargic with low testosterone and I don't sleep very well. I'm judgmental and don't try new things, which puts me on the couch a lot with distractions, vices and depression.

Write down your "Old Belief" in a Circle of Results Model.

---

2) **What are the problems created by your old belief?**

Describe the problems your old belief created – i.e., how much time was wasted, any bad habits you developed, how did you suffer, how did it make you feel?

For example: I used to waste countless hours on the couch binge watching sports and overeating ice cream. I must have wasted 5 years of my life working on other people's dreams instead of my own. I also gained a lot of weight and neglected to do anything with intensity, which limited my energy and libido and put me into a state of depression. I felt stuck, like this was going to be my life forever so I didn't take any new action.

Write Down The Problems Created by Your Old Belief

____

3) What are the benefits of your problem?

If there were a benefit to having this problem what would it be? Is there something that your unconscious mind wants you to understand that if you understood it would make the problem disappear?

For example: I realized that I was deciding to be lazy and not living up to my full potential. I didn't do much of anything with intensity, including my job, how I treated myself or how I loved others. I learned that failure from the past doesn't mean failure in the future. This new perspective allowed me to step my game up, take action and start building my intensity and immensity with the *Fired Up* program.

Write Down The Benefits Of Your Problem

____

New Belief Change Declaration #1 – Intensity Leads To Immensity

Now it's time to declare your new belief by writing it down in a Circle of Results Model and then focus on it daily.

4) How will your "New Belief" play out in a Circle of Results Model?

Example:

B – I believe laziness is just an excuse to remain stuck. I also believe that by adding intensity from a regular HIIT class I can create more immensity and feel like I'm on top of the world.   Nothing is more important than my health so I've committed to a HIIT routine for life. This brings me daily joy, maximum sexual potency and superpowers that elevate me above any challenge.

T – I think if I'm feeling slow or lazy, I can simply turn on a video from my *Fired Up* library and instantly feel on top of the world.

E – I feel excited like I really found a solution I can always count on to boost my mood and my superpowers.

A – I read the Fired Up Manual and start doing the video training.

R – Within 30 days of starting the *Fired Up* program I start to see noticeable changes in my mind and body. I feel more alive and people start to ask: "What's different about you?" They respect me more and want what I have. This gives me more confidence to take more action and pursue my passions.

Now write down a Circle of Results Model using your "New Belief":

New Belief: What do you declare as your new belief? Make sure you use Pain, Pleasure and Purpose as well as the Master Mindsets that feel most empowering to you.

____

Thought: Describe the thoughts you'll have after you've embedded this new belief.

____

Emotion: Describe how you will feel once this new belief is part of your permanent mindset.

____

____

Action: What have you been unwilling to do in order to keep this problem? Describe the action you will take which will lead to a new habit.

____

____

Result: How do you know for sure that your old belief is no longer a problem for you? Visualize your new outcome in detail – i.e., where will you be, who will be with you, any new habits created from the action, how will you feel?

Take Action

Congratulations you've just created a new empowered belief about HIIT. And since repetition is the mother of all skill, let's reflect on the importance of embedding this new belief deep into your subconscious.

In order to make this belief a more permanent part of your roots, you'll need to repeat it to yourself daily for 90 days, which will create a long-term habit.

What I recommend is you write your Circle of Results Model down in your smartphone on a notepad.

Next, open your electronic calendar and write a reminder that repeats every day for the next 90 days. All you have to do is read the note when that reminder pops up, it's really that simple.

To make it even more effective, try to memorize it and repeat it out loud to yourself.

Last but definitely not least, make absolutely sure you tell a friend or family member about your new belief and how you are committed to keeping it. This is absolutely crucial as studies show telling others about a goal helps you stay accountable and committed to upholding that belief.

Take action on this and do not hesitate. Make the call!

Different Ways To Do HIIT

Since the basic principle of HIIT is to vary high intensity with low intensity there are a multitude of ways to do it including the following:

- Plyometrics (exercises in which muscles exert maximum force in short intervals of time)
- Super Slow Strength training (as mentioned earlier)
- Calisthenics (a variety of movements which use large muscle groups)
- Cycling (indoors or outdoors)
- Rowing
- Swimming
- Sprinting

In order to teach specific techniques and various levels of difficulty, the *Fired Up* program includes videos, which focus on various options using plyometrics, calisthenics and super slow strength training. That being said, if you have an outdoor passion like cycling, swimming or climbing and would like to apply it using the principles of HIIT I recommend first reviewing the videos in the *Fired Up* program to better understand how you can apply it to your sport.

2 Categories of HIIT

There are three distinct categories of HIIT in this program, which depending on your available time and ability level, can be performed as follows:

The Nitric Oxide Dump

"Nitric Oxide Dump," is a routine that features four exercises that address your 16 major muscle groups and only requires 4 minutes to complete. Quite simply, you'll do 10 repetitions of 4 different exercises including squats, alternating arm raises, non-jumping jacks and shoulder presses without any breaks for 4 minutes 2-3 times per day (with or without weights depending on your ability level).

Dr. Zach Bush, whose triple-board certification includes expertise in internal medicine, endocrinology and metabolism, is a huge proponent of the Nitric Oxide Dump and suggests the routine works best if you complete it three times a day, waiting at least two hours between sessions, which is how long it takes for nitric oxide to synthesize in your body for subsequent release.

Says Bush, "Our blood vessels actually only store about 90 seconds worth of nitric oxide before they need to manufacture more, so working each major muscle group out for 90 seconds gives you the most efficient workout to tone and build muscles. The body has the ability to regenerate nitric oxide every couple of hours, giving you the opportunity to release it multiple times a day. What that means is the most effective way to increase your muscle function is to work out very briefly every few hours."

If you're really short on time or just don't like longer workouts the Nitric Oxide Dump could be a great routine for you.

HIIT YOGA

HIIT YOGA in the *Fired Up* Program combines the awesome benefits of both HIIT and Yoga by doing specific HIIT exercises at 70-90% of your maximum heart rate for roughly 30 to 60 seconds, then alternating with yoga postures at 60–70 % of your maximum heart rate for 1-3 minutes. This cycle of high intensity followed by low intensity is then repeated between 4 and 10 times depending on your ability level and time restrictions.

Additionally, if you have injuries or would like low impact variations, the *Fired Up* program library of videos offers both high and low impact options so anyone can do them regardless of your age or ability level.

HIIT Yoga classes take roughly 20-40 minutes to complete including warm-up and warm down and can be performed 1-3 times per week depending on intensity.

Word of Caution

Once you reach your maximum heart rate (MHR), you might feel nauseous or light headed and short of breath. Just know your body will recover quite rapidly and within 1-3 minutes, you will start to feel much better.

If you do not recover and feel overly nauseous you may have too much food in your stomach. Make sure you do NOT eat at least 2-3 hours before a HIIT class.

If food is definitely not the problem, you're more than likely feeling the nauseous effects of toxins that were previously stored in your fat cells, which are now in your bloodstream trying to leave your body through its natural detoxification process. If this is the case, slow down or stop and drink plenty of alkaline water until the nausea dissipates.

HHT Equipment

While you don't have to buy anything to do HIIT I do recommend a couple of things that can make your practice more safe and injury free.

Heart Rate Monitor

In order to get the maximum benefits from a HIIT routine, you'll need to monitor the most important factor, which is whether or not you're producing a heart rate that is close to 90% of your maximum heart rate (MHR) during the high intensity portion.

It's almost impossible to accurately measure your heart rate manually when it's above 150. Additionally, going over your maximum heart rate for your age can be dangerous and going under just isn't going to give you all the awesomeness described above. Due to these factors, I highly recommend a heart rate monitor.

Since these gadgets can easily cost hundreds of dollars, if you're on a budget I recommend just buying a chest strap, which integrates with free apps like Strava and Nike. If you're unsure which one to buy check out our resources section at www.ChadScottCoaching.com/resources

Foam Roller

If you've ever been sore before or wondered why you had aches or pains that wouldn't go away, there's a good chance it's not tension in your muscles but the tissue surrounding your muscles, otherwise known as fascia.

The best way to describe fascia is think about the casing on a sausage. This is how you're body is designed; with fascia covering just about every part of it. We mentioned how yoga helps immensely by stretching fascia but even yoga cannot address all of your fasciae.

A foam roller, on the other hand, can stretch and reduces tension in parts of your fascia yoga just can't access and it's my secret recommendation for reducing post exercise soreness.

Not only will this immediately get rid of soreness but it will take aches and pains away that you never could get rid of before. Check out my foam roller recommendation for $21 on our resources page here.

HIIT Recovery & Other Synergistic Considerations

Frequency Matters

One of the biggest reasons people give up on any type of exercise is because of the soreness after a workout, which can last several days. To reduce this soreness and recovery time make sure you employ the strategy of **"Cold Water Therapy"** mentioned in Chapter 4 and if possible buy a foam roller.

Additionally, since any kind of high intensity training takes time to recover from, we'll stick to a frequency of 1-3 times per week per muscle group maximum and skip at least 2 days between HIIT workouts.

Pay Attention to Cycles

If you're just starting out and go full blast on a HIIT class, you'll most likely be sore for a couple days. If you do not consider yourself a highly conditioned athlete, I recommend starting out with fewer cycles (4-5 instead of 8) and build up to 8 or 10.

Diet & Hydration

I highly recommended following the power building strategies from *The Power Diet* and make sure you stay hydrated with alkaline water that contains natural electrolytes. This will help disperse the build-up of lactic acid in your muscles and eliminate toxins while reducing soreness.

Music

Music is key for giving you an extra push and motivating you to complete a HIIT class. If you purchase the Fired Up online course you'll find classes with and without music. This music has been curated specifically to motivate and push you through the classes but if you would like to use your own music you can choose some upbeat playlists from Spotify by searching for "House Music" or "Exercise Playlist."

Health Disclaimer

Again, similar to strength training, by engaging in intense exercise when you're feeling unusually weak or tired you could push yourself over the edge into a state of illness. If this is the case consider a hot bath and/or some yoga instead.

Lastly, the *Fired Up* program makes no claims of medical treatment. If you have a history of heart disease or other health concerns, please get clearance from your health care professional before starting a HIIT exercise session.

THE POWER DIET - INTRODUCTION

"Let Food Be Thy Medicine and Medicine Be Thy Food" – Socrates

When it comes to optimal health and superhuman power there are several factors that could slow you down or worse, reverse your progress entirely and send you to the couch. As previously mentioned, the primary challenge is your beliefs, which not only determine whether or not you take action and get *"Fired Up"* but whether or not you decide to eat an entire pizza, a gallon of ice cream or a six pack of beer one night because you had a rough day at work or your relationships are in turmoil.

Of course, this brings us to diet or more specifically *"The Power Diet."* Once you've taken action and gotten clear on your beliefs that will create a lifelong commitment to fitness and superhuman strength you'll need to address the basics of superhuman nutrition and how this affects the success or failure of the *Fired Up* program. As such, I need to issue an important warning.

WARNING: You cannot exercise your way out of a bad diet!

This is absolutely critical and according to Doctors like Joe Mercola and Phil McGuff, your diet actually accounts for about 80 percent of the health benefits derived from a healthy lifestyle, with the remaining 20 percent coming from exercise.   Says McGuff:

"The standard American diet is highly inflammatory. It produces systemic inflammation of an order that is almost beyond belief. In that state, if you do exercise of any significant stress, you're just adding inflammation on top of the inflammation, and you're actually putting yourself at a bit of a risk. I advise people to get their diet straight and then exercise. Because I think a highly inflammatory diet, in combination with the acute systemic inflammation that occurs as a part of the exercise stimulus, can actually be a negative thing."

Further advice from Michael Mathews, best selling author of "Bigger Leaner Stronger" ads further credence to this statement by proclaiming:

"Eat wrong, and you will stay fat no matter how much cardio you do. Eat wrong, and you stay skinny and weak no matter how much you struggle with weights. Eat right, however, and you can unlock the maximum potential gains from working out: rapid, long-term fat loss and muscle growth that will turn heads and get your friends and family talking."

If you're not already hip to this, you should know that according to multiple studies, excessive inflammation is the leading cause of most major diseases including atherosclerosis, arthritis, psoriasis, gout, asthma, allergies and multiple sclerosis amongst others.[71][72] Clearly, if you're inflamed, you need to get a handle on your diet.

Fortunately, "*The Power Diet*," is derived from some of the top leading nutritionists, doctors and fitness experts in the world.

The Power Diet seamlessly integrates with the *Fired Up* program and shows you exactly what to eat, when to eat and how much to eat so you don't get bogged down in all the details.

The basic premise of the power diet relates to the timeless credo of Socrates mentioned at the very beginning of this chapter with one slight modification as follows:

"Let food be thy power and power be thy food"

In other words, if you eat according to *The Power Diet*, this food will function as powerful medicine, which will eliminate inflammation, populate your gut with super powered microbes and allow you to ditch the doctors and prescription drugs.

Most importantly, power foods give you more power, while other foods take it away. So make absolutely sure you spend a good 30 days cleaning up any inflammation that could sabotage your results from the *Fired Up* program by reading and taking action with **"The Power Diet"**. Again, I'm going to repeat myself since this is so important:

Before you workout, clean up any inflammation with *The Power Diet!*

The Power Diet Triple Threat

As the companion nutritional program to *Fired Up, The Power Diet* provides even more synergistic benefits by utilizing the power of three key elements as follows:

1) **Power Foods** – Specific foods that provide optimal energy and performance for the maximum duration of time without negative side effects.

2) **Metabolic Flexibility** – Ability to burn fat, protein and carbs with the primary fuel source being ketones from fat. This strategy creates massive benefits including reduced insulin sensitivity and autophagy, a super powered anti-aging and optimal health strategy, which allows cell waste and damaged material in your cells to be recycled into energy or new proteins.

3) **Highly Flexible Range of Macros** – Macronutrients (AKA Macros) are fat, protein and carbohydrates, which are recommended from nutritious and tasty

foods in proportions that work to naturally burn unwanted fat, build muscle, increase strength, libido and mental focus.

Together these elements create a diet that is sustainable long-term as a lifestyle, which will help you reach your most challenging goals regardless of your circumstances.

Can I Follow Another Diet?

Yes you can, just keep in mind, there are lots of other ketogenic diets on the market but most are either too complex or too strict to follow and are thus unsustainable for long-term results. In contrast, The Power Diet makes eating simple and enjoyable by showing you step by step how to build 10 minute meals that are simple to make and taste sweet, savory, delicious and fulfilling. To find out more about The Power Diet just head over to the link below.

www.ChadScottCoaching.com/power-diet

Should I Eat Before Working Out?

Eating before a workout depends on several factors including your goals, protein synthesis, and the intensity of the exercise. Let's explore some of these variables so you can maximize your return on investment.

Fat Loss

If you suffer from carrying extra poundage and would like to feel lighter on your feet with more energy one of the quickest and most effective ways to accelerate fat loss is to work out prior to your first meal of the day. If this is you just make sure and pay special attention to the "Fat Loss (Cutting)" phase later on.

Just keep in mind, if you work out in the afternoon or evening and have already eaten your first meal this most likely will not apply.

Protein Synthesis

Once you've reached your ideal weight, the next key determinant of whether or not you need to eat before you workout will be the presence or absence of protein synthesis. As mentioned in *The Power Diet*, eating protein increases muscle building (protein synthesis) and suppresses muscle breakdown rates.[73]

While the science on this subject is limited, Doctor Joe Mercola recommends eating some protein as soon as possible after a workout if you have not eaten any roughly 8 hours prior.

Intensity Of Workout

As for fat and carbohydrates, while eating them prior to working out will not lead directly to strength gains, they will improve performance and potential muscle growth, especially if your workout is intense strength training or HIIT.

For example, eating a banana 20-60 minutes before a big strength-training workout will help you push harder and may also aid in postworkout recovery and muscle growth.[74] For this reason, I recommend that you use your two days of high carb medium fat macro consumption to do your intense strength training and HIIT workouts (see *The Power Diet* for in-depth explanation).

Lastly, if you are going to eat a snack before working out, again, check *The Power Diet* snack list and if you choose something like a banana with almond butter, which includes protein, fat and carbs, you'll need to wait a good 60 minutes to digest the fat and protein.

When Should I Eat After Working Out – The Anabolic Window

While many a meathead has claimed the importance of eating right after a workout in order to raise muscle protein synthesis and hit the so called "anabolic window," this is more myth than science.

As the myth goes, you must eat within 30 minutes of working out or your body will start to break down muscle. Since your body only builds muscle when your rates of muscle protein synthesis (MPS) are greater than your rates of muscle protein breakdown (MPD) this is important. But in reality, studies show that muscle protein breakdown is only slightly raised post-workout.[75]

Adding another nail in the coffin to the anabolic window myth is a meta study conducted by bodybuilding researchers Alan Aragon and Brad Schoenfeld who concluded that there is "zero conclusive evidence that shows ingesting carbs and protein immediately after a workout raises muscle protein synthesis." [76]

Essentially, you don't need to worry about eating within this mythical 30-minute anabolic window, but you do need to eat at some point.

So here's the deal: if you haven't eaten in over 24-48 hours, you will eventually run out of glucose and ketones with nothing for your body to draw on for energy. At this point, your body will begin breaking down muscle tissue – not a good thing. Of course, with the exception of an extended fast, this will be a rare occasion.

A more likely scenario is eating dinner at 7pm, going to sleep, then working out in a fasted state at around 9am. In this case, studies show that muscle protein breakdown is significantly raised post-workout.[77] For this reason, it is strongly advised that if you have not eaten protein within the last 4-6 hours after a workout you should eat as soon as possible, otherwise, you could be breaking down (catabolic) muscle when you should be building it (anabolic).

Special Note On Fasted Workouts – While working out in a fasted state can burn fat quickly and expedite your transition to metabolic flexibility, if you are not yet metabolically flexible you'll want to workout shortly after waking up as you could experience some serious fatigue if you wait too long.   Make sure you read *The Power Diet* for further instructions on fasted workouts and what power foods to eat for maximum strength and power.

www.ChadScottCoaching.com/power-diet

CHAPTER 7 – SUPERPOWERED WORKOUT ROUTINES

"Nothing in this world can take the place of persistence. Talent will not; nothing is more common than unsuccessful men with talent. Genius will not; unrewarded genius is almost a proverb. Education will not; the world is full of educated derelicts. Persistence and determination alone are omnipotent. The slogan Press On! has solved and always will solve the problems of the human race." - Calvin Coolidge (30th President of the United States of America)

Now that you're on target with *The Power Diet* and have removed unwanted inflammation, it's time to "Press On" and continue stacking the deck in your favor by answering the following question:

What Is My Current State Of Fitness?

This is highly significant since reaching your goal of optimum health and superhuman power requires that you choose just the right workout program for your current fitness level.

If for instance, you choose a program that focuses on maintaining a high level of fitness but you're overweight or over inflamed you could injure yourself, get frustrated or just give up because you don't get quick results.

To avoid this pitfall and reach an optimal fitness level your first goal will be to reset your body to its ideal weight.

Once you achieve your ideal weight with both *Fired Up* and *The Power Diet*, your body won't have to work so hard carrying around extra poundage and your natural powers of hormone regulation, detoxification, immunity, sexual potency and superhuman strength, will restore themselves naturally. To get to this point, first, you need to answer another question as follows:

What Is My Ideal Body Weight?

To determine if you are at the proper weight is more intuition than science. As such, we'll need to investigate a little further with another question:

When Did You Last Feel You Were At Your Ideal Weight?

For many people, the answer to this question was high school or college when you were more active. But if you think about this logically, unless you're pregnant or training to be a bodybuilder or professional athlete, there is no healthy reason to gain more weight after you've filled out your frame and stopped growing in height.

As for science, one of the standard measurements of correct weight is your BMI or Body Mass Index.

Health practitioners use BMI to estimate body fat and possible health risks related to weight. This is important, especially if you've struggled with being overweight and you don't know what your ideal weight is.

To calculate your BMI and ideal weight literally takes 30 seconds. Just follow this link to find out then come right back: https://chadscottcoaching.com/bmi

Factor In Your Body Type

Question: Did your BMI fall between 18.5 and 24.9? According to the National Heart, Lung and Blood Institute, this is considered a healthy range for ideal body weight. Unfortunately, it's not an exact science, as it doesn't take into consideration your body type. To get more accurate let's check out the three basic body types and their ideal BMI as follows:

Ectomorphic - Long, lean and thin defines the Ectomorphic body type. If this is you, you most likely have trouble putting muscle on your small frame and have challenges gaining weight, no matter how much you eat. When measuring your BMI your ideal weight should fall in the lower ranges closer to 18.5.

Endomorphic - If this is you, you're the opposite of an Ectomorph and you'll have larger bones with a fuller figure. If this is you, you'll most likely gain weight easily, have a large bone structure and experience challenges creating muscle definition. When measuring your BMI your ideal weight should fall in the upper ranges around the 24.9 mark.

Mesomorphic - If this is you, you're in the middle and will tend to gain muscle fairly easily. When following good nutrition and exercise, you'll usually have wide shoulders, a small waist, a medium bone structure and low body fat. When measuring your BMI your ideal weight should fall in the mid-range around 21.

Again, to measure your BMI in under 30 seconds just follow the link below then come back to determine the best workout plan for you. https://chadscottcoaching.com/bmi

The 3 Workout Programs

After you've determined your ideal weight, you'll need to pick one of the following routines based on whether or not you're overweight, underweight or at your ideal weight.

1) **Fat Loss (Cutting Phase) 12 Week Program:** If you are overweight by more than 10 pounds I recommend focusing on the "Cutting" phase first. This will place a heavy focus on burning off excess fat to restore your body's natural healing and strengthening powers.   If you combine

the food recommendations from *The Power Diet* with this program you should get pretty close to your ideal weight within 3-6 months; if not, just keep going until you do. Once you achieve your ideal weight go ahead and switch to the "Maintenance & Expansion" program.

2) **Weight Gain 12 Week Program:** If you are underweight and need more muscle I recommend this phase, which will focus on minimizing fat gain with less HIIT and more carbs. Once you achieve your ideal weight on this program go ahead and switch to the "Maintenance & Expansion" program.

3) **Maintenance & Expansion (M&E):** This program is designed as the ultimate goal of the *Fired Up* program. To be clear, this is not a stagnant, stay the same routine. Rather, this is a lifestyle change, which will continue to create optimum health and maximum power for the duration of your life.

Can I Lose Weight on Maintenance & Expansion?

I often get asked this question from clients who don't want to cut carbs and increase their weekly HIIT. The short answer is "Yes" you can lose weight by following the Maintenance & Expansion program. The only difference is that Maintenance &

Expansion will simply take longer to lose weight than the cutting program.

So if you're ok with potentially doubling the time it takes to get to your ideal weight, then, by all means, skip the Fat Loss program and start with Maintenance & Expansion.

Let's go ahead and break down each of the three programs one by one.

Maintenance & Expansion Program (M&E)

As the cornerstone of the *Fired Up* program, "Maintenance & Expansion" is what separates the boys from the men, the girls from the women, and… this program from most other workout programs.

Essentially, instead of shifting from weight loss to weight gain like a never-ending rollercoaster, the "Maintenance & Expansion" program combined with *The Power Diet* gives your body just the right fuel and function to maintain optimal health while continuing to expand and fine-tune your mental, physical and spiritual power.

Recommended Food Consumption for M&E

In *Fired Up* and *The Power Diet*, we don't recommend counting calories as this strategy is not only a pain in the ass but rarely works. Make sure you follow *The Power Diet* recommendations and video library for making meals, optimizing performance and building superhuman power.

Time For Action

To make this initial leap into *The Power Diet* as painless as possible you'll need to take the recommended actions so pay close attention to the following:

You Are Your Habits

You've most likely heard the phrase "We are creatures of habit." This is super important and critical to your success, for without a long-term habit you'll eventually fall prey to the call of your couch and a bag of potato chips.

The Fired Up program will guide you day by day on what action to take for 90 days. But this is by no means determined by the random toss of a dart. In fact, research led by a team at the University College London found it takes, on average, 66 days to form a habit.

Essentially, by taking the recommended actions for a good 90 days you'll have created one of the best habits imaginable, which will support you for the rest of your life.

At this point, you'll be on autopilot without having to think much about getting "*Fired Up*;" this is where the real magic starts to happen. Where your life transforms with more abundance in health, wealth, loving relationships and pure joy. To do this I recommend two primary strategies as follows:

Option 1 – Video Library Daily Check In

Option 1 is my ideal recommendation and can be achieved by checking in daily with the 90 day *Fired Up* online video library. This will guide you day-by-day as to what actions you need to take in order to optimize for maximum performance and power while creating a habit that will serve you for the rest of your life.

Just keep in mind, this doesn't mean you'll be grinding it out every day of the week with a full class. Instead, you'll have 4-5 days on and 2-3 days off each week depending on which program you choose.

Option 2 - Video Library 3-Day Minimum Check In

While the day-by-day Option 1 program is ideal, your schedule may change from week to week and this simply may not work. If you need to be more flexible with your schedule (i.e. you're traveling, get injured or sick) you can stick to the minimum by completing at least 3 classes per week. If you choose this route you'll need to check in to the *Fired Up* video library at least three days per week and pick a class from each of our 3 synergistic categories as follows:

- STRENGTH TRAINING - 1 Day
- YOGA - 1 Day
- HIIT YOGA - 1 Day

Regardless of whether you choose Option 1 or 2, make sure you opt in to the 90 day reminder which will send you an email every day to not only remind you of the class for the day but to encourage and motivate you to keep going. To learn more how the video program works check out the link below.

www.chadscottcoaching.com/fired-up-lifetime

Fired Up M&E Training - Weeks 1-4

Keep in mind; while M&E will be a program you can do for the rest of your life, I've created a 90-day introduction, which will allow you to explore the different possibilities for weekly workouts.

Essentially, what you do on each day and what time you do it will be based on your own personal preference and circumstances.

If for example, you're just wiped out on Mondays you may need to make yoga your first class of the week and build up to strength training and HIIT. If you do need to change the recommended schedule just make sure you at least complete "Option 2 - Three Day Minimum Check In" as noted above.

Make sure you experiment with the different recommended routines to find out which works best for your personal circumstances. Now let's check out the weekly schedule for the Maintenance & Expansion program.

Monday	Strength Training or SST (Full Body Push, Pull, Legs)

	Push Barbell or Dumbbell Bench Press 3 Sets 4-8 Reps Overhead Dumbbell Press 3 Sets 4-8 Reps **Pull** Chinups, Pullups or Lat Pulldown 3 Sets 4-8 Reps **Legs** Squats or Bulgarian Split Lunges 3 Sets 4-8 Reps **No Weights Option -** Watch Strength Training Videos
Tuesday	Yoga 30-60 minute class
Wednesday	HIIT Yoga or Nitric Oxide Dump
Thursday	Breathwork, Walk or Fun Activity Outdoors
Friday	Yoga 1 hour class
Saturday	Yoga (Restorative) or Fun Activity
Sunday	Breathwork, Rest, Walk or Fun Activity Outdoors

Special Note on HIIT categories: If you struggle with some of the more advanced HIIT routines offered due to age, injury or medical condition, feel free to lower the intervals or substitute with:

1) Nitric Oxide Dump

2) Super Slow Strength Training

Fired Up M&E Training - Week 5-8

During your second 30 days in M&E you can continue on the same schedule or begin adding in some isolation exercises and adding or subtracting from each of the three synergistic elements Yoga, HIIT or Strength Training.

Below is a suggested routine, which splits Strength Training into two separate days (upper body and lower body) and adds in some isolation exercises. Again, this is just a suggestion but if you have challenges with shoulder and knee joints or just want to up your game another level, I recommend giving this a shot.

Alternatively, you could simply stick to your previous routine with one full body Strength Training day (push, pull, legs) but simply combine the two days into one longer workout.

If you decide to change it up on the second 30 days, again just make sure you at least complete "Option 2 - Three Day Minimum Check In."

Lastly, this 4-week period should also follow the 8-week drawdown as outlined in *The Power Diet*.

Monday	**Strength Training or SST (Push, Pull, Isolation)**
	Push

	Dumbbell or Barbell Bench Press 2-3 Sets 4-8 Reps Overhead Dumbbell Press 2-3 Sets 4-8 Reps **Pull** Chin Ups 2 Sets 4-8 Reps Pull Ups 2 Sets 4-8 Reps Curls 2 Sets 4-8 Reps **Shoulder Isolation** Lateral Raise 2 sets 8-15 Reps Frontal Raise 2 sets 8-15 Reps Angled Raise 2 sets 8-15 Reps **No Weights Option -** Watch Strength Training Videos
Tuesday	Yoga 30-60 minute class
Wednesday	HIIT Yoga or Nitric Oxide Dump
Thursday	Breathwork, Yoga, Walk or Fun Activity Outdoors
Friday	**Strength Training or SST (Legs, Core)** **Legs** Forward Lunge 2 Sets 8-15 Reps Side Lunge slide 2 Sets 8-15 Reps Squat 2-3 Sets 4-8 Reps Dead Lift 2-3 Sets 4-8 Reps

	Core Core Leg Lifts 3 Sets 5-15 Reps **No Weights Option -** Watch Strength Training Videos
Saturday	Yoga (Restorative) or Fun Activity
Sunday	Breathwork, Rest, Walk or Fun Activity Outdoors

Fired Up M&E Training - Week 9-12

In your final 30 days of exploring the M&E program, you should be finding your groove in a workout that works best for your personal circumstances. That being said, I'll offer one additional option to mix things up and make sure you have the most optimal routine for building superhuman power.

The program below adds in one big Strength Training day and an additional HIIT Yoga day, which will challenge you to the max. So be forewarned, if this is beyond your capability or you find it takes a long time to recover simply back off and reduce your frequency with more time off for rest and recovery.

Monday	Strength Training or SST (Push, Pull, Legs)
	Push Dumbbell or Barbell Bench Press 2-3 Sets 4-8 Reps Overhead Dumbbell Press 2-3 Sets 4-8 Reps **Pull** Chin Ups 2 Sets 4-8 Reps Curls 2 Sets 4-8 Reps **Legs** Forward Lunge 2 Sets 8-15 Reps

	Side Lunge side 2 Sets 8-15 Reps Squat 2-3 Sets 4-8 Reps Dead Lift 2-3 Sets 4-8 Reps **Core** Core Leg Lifts 3 Sets 5-15 Reps **Shoulders** Lateral Raise 2 sets 8-15 Reps Frontal Raise 2 sets 8-15 Reps Angled Raise 2 sets 8-15 Reps **No Weights Option -** Watch Strength Training Videos
Tuesday	Yoga 60 minute class
Wednesday	HIIT Yoga or Nitric Oxide Dump
Thursday	Breathwork, Walk or Fun Activity Outdoors
Friday	HIIT Yoga or Nitric Oxide Dump
Saturday	Yoga (Restorative) or Fun Activity
Sunday	Breathwork, Rest, Walk or Fun Activity Outdoors

Fat Loss (Cutting Phase) - 12 Week Program

For the most part, the fat loss or cutting phase stays the same as the M&E program over the first 12 weeks with the following modifications:

1) **Shorter eating window** - You will gradually decrease your eating window from 10 to 6 hours. Make sure you follow *The Power Diet* 8-week drawdown.

2) **Less Carbs** – You will eat less carbs (5-15% of your total macros). Again, make sure you follow *The Power Diet* recommendations.

3) **Increase HIIT frequency** – By increasing your HIIT intervals every 30 days, the "Cutting Phase" will unlock fat deposits and shed unwanted weight much faster. Just make sure you pay attention to the highlighted changes as you finish each 30-day period. Also, keep in mind, if you feel the HIIT intervals are just too much for your ability level, back off and stick with the prior weeks' recommendation until you feel ready to advance.

Best Time To Exercise For Weight Loss

By exercising before your first meal, you'll increase your fat burning power multiplicatively. This massive benefit is detailed in *The Power Diet* and explains how becoming metabolically flexible increases your overall power and efficiency.

Multiple studies confirm that when employing a low carbohydrate, high fat diet, the oxidation of fat is increased during exercise, especially during a HIIT class.

For example, one study found that in subjects who restricted carbohydrates and increased fat consumption, up to 70% of their energy requirements (even during high intensity activities) came from the oxidation of fat. [78]

In contrast, in a high carb diet, such activities would derive 80-90% of the energy from glycogen. [79]

Essentially, by working out before you eat, you'll begin to train your body to burn fat as it's primary fuel source and not only will you burn off ugly unwanted fat but eventually end overwhelming cravings for carbohydrates.

Skipping breakfast and instead, working out is one of the power strategies mentioned in *The Power Diet* and will be a game changer for achieving your ideal weight and boosting your power to maximum. Again, if you're not already clear about why this is so important, make sure you review *The Power Diet* and get really clear before moving on.

Minimum Weekly Workouts

While you can do more than the suggested weekly minimum, make sure you at least complete the following each week:

- HIIT YOGA - 2 Days
- Strength Training – 1 Day

*   Yoga - 1 Day

Fired Up Weight Loss Phase - Weeks 1-4

Below is a recommendation of daily workouts for your first 30 days on the Weight Loss Phase. Remember, this is a flexible program; as long as you're hitting the minimum requirements, feel free to switch any of these workouts to a different day if it makes more sense for your personal schedule.

Additionally, if you struggle with some of the more advanced HIIT routines offered due to age, injury or medical condition, feel free to lower the intervals or substitute with the Nitric Oxide Dump or SST.

Monday	**Strength Training or SST (Full Body Push, Pull, Legs)** **Push** Barbell or Dumbbell Bench Press 3 Sets 4-8 Reps Overhead Dumbbell Press 3 Sets 4-8 Reps **Pull** Chinups, Pullups or Lat Pulldown 3 Sets 4-8 Reps **Legs** Squats or Bulgarian Split Lunges 3 Sets 4-8 Reps

	No Weights Option - Watch Strength Training Videos
Tuesday	Yoga 30-60 minute class
Wednesday	HIIT Yoga or Nitric Oxide Dump
Thursday	Breathwork, Walk or Fun Activity Outdoors
Friday	HIIT Yoga or Nitric Oxide Dump
Saturday	Yoga (Restorative) or Fun Activity
Sunday	Breathwork, Rest, Walk or Fun Activity Outdoors

Fired Up Weight Loss Phase - Weeks 5-8

During your second 30 days, you can continue on the same schedule or begin adding in some isolation exercises and adding or subtracting from each of the three synergistic elements Yoga, HIIT or Strength Training.

Below is a suggested routine, which adds in some isolation exercises to your Strength Training day. Again, this is just a suggestion but if you have challenges with shoulder and knee joints or just want to up your game another level, I recommend giving this a shot.

If you decide to change it up on the second 30 days, again just make sure you at least complete "Option 2 - Three Day Minimum Check In."

Lastly, this 4-week period should also follow the 8-week drawdown as outlined in *The Power Diet*.

Monday	Strength Training or SST (Push, Pull, Legs) **Push** Dumbbell or Barbell Bench Press 2-3 Sets 4-8 Reps Overhead Dumbbell Press 2-3 Sets 4-8 Reps **Pull** Chin Ups 2 Sets 4-8 Reps Curls 2 Sets 4-8 Reps **Legs** Forward Lunge 2 Sets 8-15 Reps Side Lunge side 2 Sets 8-15 Reps Squat 2-3 Sets 4-8 Reps Dead Lift 2-3 Sets 4-8 Reps **Core** Core Leg Lifts 3 Sets 5-15 Reps **Shoulders** Lateral Raise 2 sets 8-15 Reps Frontal Raise 2 sets 8-15 Reps

	Angled Raise 2 sets 8-15 Reps **No Weights Option -** Watch Strength Training Videos
Tuesday	Yoga 30-60 minute class
Wednesday	HIIT Yoga or Nitric Oxide Dump
Thursday	Breathwork, Walk or Fun Activity Outdoors
Friday	HIIT Yoga or Nitric Oxide Dump
Saturday	Yoga (Restorative) or Fun Activity
Sunday	Breathwork, Rest, Walk or Fun Activity Outdoors

Fired Up Weight Loss Phase - Week 9-12

In your final 30 days of the Fired Up Weight Loss Phase, you should be feeling lighter, happier and more powerful as that poundage starts to melt off. At this point, you can continue with either of the programs from the 1st or 2nd 30 days just make sure you place special emphasis on three things as follows:

1) Increase your intervals of HIIT YOGA. For example, if you could only do 4 intervals try 6 or 8.
2) Try working out before you've eaten your first meal.

3) Reduce your carbohydrate consumption to 5-10% of your total caloric intake (see *The Power Diet* for further clarification)

The program below is simply a repeat of your 2nd 30-day routine. Make absolutely sure you are honest with yourself about expectations. If this routine is beyond your capability or you find it takes a long time to recover simply back off and reduce your frequency with more time off for rest and recovery.

Monday	Strength Training or SST (Push, Pull, Legs) **Push** Dumbbell or Barbell Bench Press 2-3 Sets 4-8 Reps Overhead Dumbbell Press 2-3 Sets 4-8 Reps **Pull** Chin Ups 2 Sets 4-8 Reps Curls 2 Sets 4-8 Reps **Legs** Forward Lunge 2 Sets 8-15 Reps Side Lunge side 2 Sets 8-15 Reps Squat 2-3 Sets 4-8 Reps Dead Lift 2-3 Sets 4-8 Reps

	Core
	Core Leg Lifts 3 Sets 5-15 Reps
	Shoulders
	Lateral Raise 2 sets 8-15 Reps
	Frontal Raise 2 sets 8-15 Reps
	Angled Raise 2 sets 8-15 Reps
	No Weights Option - Watch Strength Training Videos
Tuesday	Yoga 60 minute class
Wednesday	HIIT Yoga or Nitric Oxide Dump
Thursday	Breathwork, Walk or Fun Activity Outdoors
Friday	HIIT Yoga or Nitric Oxide Dump
Saturday	Yoga (Restorative) or Fun Activity
Sunday	Breathwork, Rest, Walk or Fun Activity Outdoors

Once you finish your 12-week program if you have not achieved your ideal weight, continue on this same program until you do. Once you achieve your ideal weight go ahead and switch to the M&E program.

Weight Gain - 12 Week Program

If you are under your ideal weight by 10 pounds or more you may suffer from various challenges ranging from malnutrition to depression to muscle wasting. Since I can't give you an exact diagnosis, you'll need to be really honest about where you're at and potentially seek a professional diagnosis.

Regardless of your underlying condition multiple studies like the ones already mentioned, show the building of muscle to be beneficial for your health. But in order to build muscle and fill in your frame you'll need to take into consideration the following modifications:

1) **Additional Calories** – In order to gain weight, you'll need to eat more calories. Since muscle is denser than fat, (1 cup muscle = 9.7 oz. vs. 1 cup of fat = 7.5 oz.), by replacing unwanted fat with muscle you can increase your overall weight much more effectively. As mentioned in *The Power Diet*, eating protein increases muscle building (protein synthesis) and suppresses muscle breakdown rates. Accordingly, you'll need to eat more protein. And while *The Power Diet* does not focus on carbohydrates as a primary fuel source, you will need a moderate increase in carbohydrate consumption as well. To simplify this process, shoot for adding in a couple snacks from *The Power Diet* in between meals or increasing the percentage of food in your regular meals by 15-20%.

2) **Longer Eating Window** – While we will continue to deemphasize eating with high frequency, the eating window in the weight gain phase will remain in a generous range of 9-10 hours in order to accommodate the extra calories needed to be consumed.

3) **Decrease HIIT frequency** – Since HIIT burns fat faster than the other disciplines, we'll moderate this activity to once per week.

4) **Increase Strength Training with Less Reps** – As mentioned previously, studies show that strength training with less reps creates more bulk.[80] Accordingly, this program recommends more strength training days using more weight with less reps (4-6 on most exercises).

Side Note For The Ladies: As mentioned previously, if you're a woman looking to increase your weight you will not need to worry about becoming bulky. The bulk comes primarily from higher testosterone levels found only in men. That being said, focus on keeping your reps in the moderate range (6-8 instead of 4-6). This will help ensure the building of a lean, rather than a bulky physique.

Best Time To Exercise For Weight Gain

Unlike the weight loss program, which expedites fat loss by exercising in a fasted state, in the weight gain program you can workout after breakfast or any other meal. Just make sure if you consume protein or fat to eat it at least 1-2 hours prior to your workout for proper digestion. Carbohydrates like bananas, on the other hand, can be eaten in as little as 20 minutes prior to your workout.

For example, if you haven't eaten protein in the three to four hours prior to working out, then I recommend eating 30 to 40 grams before you start. On the other hand, if you've already eaten protein within that 3-4 hour range, current scientific evidence does not support additional strength or muscle gains through supplementation prior to working out.[81]

Minimum Weekly Workouts

While you can do more than the suggested weekly minimum, make sure you at least complete the following each week:

- HIIT - 1 Day
- Strength Training – 2 Days
- Yoga - 1 Day

Fired Up Weight Gain Phase - Weeks 1-4

Now let's break down the weight gain program week by week. Take a note of the changes that add or subtract from the previous programs.

Monday	**Strength Training or SST (Push, Pull)** **Push** Dumbbell or Barbell Bench Press 2-3 Sets 4-8 Reps Overhead Dumbbell Press 2-3 Sets 4-8 Reps **Pull** Chin Ups 2 Sets 4-8 Reps Curls 2 Sets 4-8 Reps **Shoulders** Lateral Raise 2 sets 8-15 Reps Frontal Raise 2 sets 8-15 Reps Angled Raise 2 sets 8-15 Reps **No Weights Option -** Watch Strength Training Videos
Tuesday	Yoga 60 minute class
Wednesday	HIIT Yoga or Nitric Oxide Dump
Thursday	Breathwork, Walk or Fun Activity Outdoors
Friday	**Strength Training or SST (Legs, Core)**

	Legs
	Forward Lunge 2 Sets 8-15 Reps
	Side Lunge side 2 Sets 8-15 Reps
	Squat 2-3 Sets 4-8 Reps
	Dead Lift 2-3 Sets 4-8 Reps
	Core
	Core Leg Lifts 3 Sets 5-15 Reps
Saturday	Yoga (Restorative) or Fun Activity
Sunday	Breathwork, Rest, Walk or Fun Activity Outdoors

Fired Up Weight Gain Phase - Weeks 5-8

In your second 30-day period in the Weight Gain Phase, you can continue on with the same routine or mix it up with a variety of strategies. For example, if you prefer to shorten your Strength Training days you can do two full body days with shorter routines as follows:

Monday	**Strength Training or SST (Full Body Push, Pull, Legs)**
	Push
	Barbell or Dumbbell Bench Press 3 Sets 4-8 Rep

	Overhead Dumbbell Press 3 Sets 4-8 Reps **Pull** Chinups, Pullups or Lat Pulldown 3 Sets 4-8 Reps **Legs** Squats or Bulgarian Split Lunges 3 Sets 4-8 Reps **No Weights Option -** Watch Strength Training Videos
Tuesday	Yoga 30-60 minute class
Wednesday	HIIT Yoga or Nitric Oxide Dump
Thursday	Breathwork, Walk or Fun Activity Outdoors
Friday	**Strength Training or SST (Full Body Push, Pull, Legs)** **Push** Barbell or Dumbbell Bench Press 3 Sets 4-8 Rep Overhead Dumbbell Press 3 Sets 4-8 Reps **Pull** Chinups, Pullups or Lat Pulldown 3 Sets 4-8 Reps **Legs** Squats 3 Sets 4-8 Reps

	No Weights Option - Watch Strength Training Videos
Saturday	Breathwork, Yoga (Restorative) or Fun Activity
Sunday	Rest, Walk or Fun Activity Outdoors

Fired Up Weight Gain Phase - Weeks 9-12

In your final 30-day period in the Weight Gain Phase, you should be filling out your frame and feeling really strong. At this point, you can continue on with the same routine or boost your Strength Training days with a full workout on both days.

Make absolutely sure you are honest with yourself about expectations. If this routine is beyond your capability or you find it takes a long time to recover simply back off and reduce your frequency with more time off for rest and recovery.

Lastly, you'll need to continue adding in an additional 15-20% boost in calories as outlined in *The Power Diet*.

Monday	**Strength Training or SST (Push, Pull, Legs)** **Push** Dumbbell or Barbell Bench Press 2-3 Sets 4-8 Reps Overhead Dumbbell Press 2-3 Sets 4-8 Reps

	Pull Chin Ups 2 Sets 4-8 Reps Curls 2 Sets 4-8 Reps **Legs** Forward Lunge 2 Sets 8-15 Reps Side Lunge side 2 Sets 8-15 Reps Squat 2-3 Sets 4-8 Reps Dead Lift 2-3 Sets 4-8 Reps **Core** Core Leg Lifts 3 Sets 5-15 Reps **Shoulders** Lateral Raise 2 sets 8-15 Reps Frontal Raise 2 sets 8-15 Reps Angled Raise 2 sets 8-15 Reps **No Weights Option -** Watch Strength Training Videos
Tuesday	Yoga 60 minute class
Wednesday	HIIT Yoga or Nitric Oxide Dump
Thursday	Breathwork, Walk or Fun Activity Outdoors
Friday	Strength Training or SST - Same as Monday

| Saturday | Yoga (Restorative) or Fun Activity |
| Sunday | Breathwork, Rest, Walk or Fun Activity Outdoors |

If you have yet to reach your ideal weight (within 10 pounds) after 12 weeks in the Weight Gain phase continue on until you do. Once you are within 10 pounds of your ideal weight it's time to switch to the Maintenance and Expansion program for the long-term.

CHAPTER 8 – TYING IT ALL TOGETHER

First off congratulations on making it this far. Most people never finish the books or the trainings they buy and you my friend are unique in that regard. So take a moment to just savor the fact that you already show signs of superhuman powers and now it's time to expand on them.

While this may be the end of the *Fired Up* Manual, it's really just the beginning of building superhuman power. To really get "Fired Up" and make serious changes in your life you'll need to do one thing over and above anything else. Now can you guess what that is?

If you guessed take action, you're right!

Take Action – Get Started Now!

Remember, without action, you simply won't get any new results. Make sure you take action right now and get started by following these steps:

Step 1) Get *The Power Diet*

Remember, you can't work your way out of a bad diet and your diet represents upwards of 80% of your total health.

Think of your mind and body like a fine tuned Ferrari; they both need high-octane fuel and when you dump low-grade fuel like

French fries and sugar cookies in it, things start to shut down and eventually it blows up.

Right now it's time to step into your new Ferrari! So if you don't already own *The Power Diet* head over to the following link and grab a copy:

www.ChadScottCoaching.com/Power-Diet

Step 2) Visit The Fired Up Video Library

This program has a full video library of classes that guide you step-by-step through the three synergistic elements of HIIT, Yoga, and Strength Training. Again, you can follow Option 1 by checking in each day and following along or follow Option 2 by completing the minimum classes, as previously suggested.

To get a 25% discount on the Fired Up Video Program just use discount code: "Firedup-25-off-readers-only" and follow the link below:

https://chadscottcoaching.com/fired-up-lifetime/

Step 3) Set A Non-Negotiable Goal

If for any reason you believe goals are a waste of time, you may as well just throw in the towel and give up now.

Really, if you just think about all the times you told yourself or someone else you needed to take action on something important and never followed through I'd wager you'd be able to recall at least a few missed opportunities.

The real question here is why didn't you take action? Could it be that you simply didn't believe it was that important and you were not fully committed to take the action necessary to make it happen?

Unfortunately, without action, your desires and goals are just dreams you'll take with you to the grave. But when you set a "Non-Negotiable Goal" by writing it down, sharing it with others and scheduling it in your calendar, you'll have a much better chance at achieving that goal.

So think of this non-negotiable goal as an unbreakable pact with yourself, something that you must do or else your entire life will be a complete waste of time.

For instance, would you have any regrets if you made food more important than anything else in your life and as a result died overweight at an early age, instead of cultivating loving relationships with your family or working on your dreams?

Would you have any regrets if you spent your whole life sedentary, overweight, or injured, which eventually killed you with a virus or fatal heart disease?

Now just take a minute to re-read those two scenarios and really feel the pain of regret. This is really important because it helps you get leverage over the weak minded lesser you that isn't willing to take the action necessary to really step up and cut the chains of laziness.

Next, after you've read those scenarios and really felt how important it is to take control of your health do you now feel a stronger commitment to taking action on *the Fired Up program*?

I'm going to assume that's a big "Yes," which means it's time to get serious and feed your Ferrari with some high-octane fuel. To do this you'll need to ask yourself the following question:

What do I need most when it comes to exercise?

There are typically two obvious goals here. The first of which is to simply lose weight. If this is you, you'll want to set a goal to lose 50% of your target weight loss within 1-3 months and the other 50% in another 1-3 months.

So let's say you're 50 pounds overweight and you set a goal to lose 25 pounds in 3 months with an additional 25 pounds in another 3 months. Since 50 pounds is a good chunk of fat and losing too much weight too quickly (more than 2 pounds per week) can put you at risk of many health problems, including muscle loss, gallstones and nutritional deficiencies, this goal can realistically be achieved by simply sticking to *Fired Up* and *The Power Diet*. [82] [83]

In contrast, if you are 20 pounds overweight you could more easily create a goal of losing 10 pounds in 1-2 months and an additional 10 pounds in another 1-2 months.

The next most common goal I find is to simply increase strength and feel powerful or solve a health issue like back pain, insulin resistance or arthritis. If this is you, I recommend setting your goal to get through the 90-day program and make your new fitness program a lifetime habit.

To get clear on what a non-negotiable goal would look like for you let's take a look at a few examples:

Weight Loss

I am committed to losing 16 pounds in 8 weeks and will take all the action steps in *Fired Up* by scheduling them in my calendar and following through. Taking these actions is non-negotiable! I am 100% committed to my health and will not break my pact with myself no matter what the circumstances are!

Health Issue

I am committed to getting rid of my back pain and will take all the action steps in *Fired Up* by scheduling them in my calendar and following through. Taking these actions is non-negotiable! I am 100% committed to my health and will not break my pact with myself no matter what the circumstances!

Feeling Stronger with More Power

I am committed to feeling better with more power and energy. I will take all the action steps in *Fired Up* by scheduling them in my calendar and following through. Taking these actions is non-negotiable! I am 100% committed to my health and will not break my pact with myself no matter what the circumstances!

NOTE: While that 100% commitment statement at the end may sound a bit rigid, just remember *Fired Up* is not rigid, it's flexible and allows you to change your routine and have fun moving your body. The commitment here is simply to stick to the 90-day *Fired Up* program and create a lifetime habit.

Write Down Your Non-Negotiable Goal Now!

Now go ahead and take action by writing down your non-negotiable goal and placing it somewhere you can see it every day like your kitchen or bathroom. I suggest printing this out and framing it in a plastic frame like this one from Amazon, which only costs a few dollars.

Step 4) – Get Accountability & Support

Taking action on the first three steps is a great start but you'll need to take one more crucial step if you are to fully commit and take the necessary action to create a lifetime habit. This brings us to the final piece of the commitment puzzle - accountability! As personal development master Jim Rohn once said:

> **"You are the average of the five people you spend the most time with?"**

Adding to this wise perspective is Jim's most successful mentee Tony Robbins who declared:

> **"Most people's lives are a direct reflection of**
> **the expectations of their peer group."**

Yes, you'll need to make an effort to surround yourself with people who are also trying to improve themselves or in the business of self-improvement. And if you're at all doubtful of this advice consider the accountability study we mentioned earlier by The American Society of Training and Development (ASTD).

In this study, researchers found that you have a 65% chance of completing a goal if you commit to someone. Additionally, if you have a specific accountability appointment with a person you've committed, you will increase your chance of success by up to 95%.[84]

To stay on track and push through the

inevitable minefields along the way, you'll need to actively seek out people to surround yourself with who are trying to improve their health or are interested in your health. These people, which could also be coaches, teachers, and mentors, will help you stay on track by supporting you with encouragement, experience and knowledge no single teacher could ever provide.

They'll also help in holding you accountable, which will give you a much-needed push when you lose motivation and things seem hopeless.

Let's face it; in the beginning, when you're excited about feeling good, you'll probably take some action for the first few weeks. But four, five or ten weeks down the road, if you don't have the motivation, discipline and accountability to stay on track, you may just sink into a comfortable couch and gorge yourself on power draining foods.

To avoid this trap, you'll need to take action right now by finding an accountability partner. Go ahead and **call or text someone** who cares about your health and tell them about your non-negotiable goal.

We'll talk more about accountability in a moment but for now, this is the simplest thing you can do to get accountability.

Text or Call your accountability partner now!

Step 5) The Next Level

If you have any questions or challenges implementing *Fired Up* or *The Power Diet* and making them a long-term lifestyle just know, I got your back!

If for any reason you feel challenged to implement these action steps or feel like your level of discipline just can't support the transformation, I'd like to invite you to check out my intelligent accountability coaching and online trainings for boosting your brain and body to maximum power and living up to your full potential.

This includes *Fired Up* and *The Power Diet*, which work synergistically to accelerate the building of a powerful, strong, and flexible mind and body. You can find out more info on this program by following this link:

https://chadscottcoaching.com/contact/

If you struggle with discipline and taking action, I recommend one of the most powerful brain building programs ever created called "The Winner's Mindset."

This powerful audio program uses advanced neurological repatterning techniques to help you embed the mindsets of over 175 masters from sports, business, politics, arts, science, medicine and spirituality.

The Winner's Mindset took me over 10 years to create and it's my most trusted source for guaranteed results in all areas of life including increasing your wealth, finding love, building relationships and boosting your health to superhuman. To get a 50%

discount use code: "WM-BookReadersOnly-50%-off" at checkout. To find out more visit the following link:

https://chadscottcoaching.com/wm-ss-sales/

With that, I'd like to congratulate you. You're now in the top 5% of the world's population, doing things most would never even imagine doing. And… you're well on your way to building a habit that will support your health and boost your power for the rest of your life.
    Just make absolutely sure you take action on those top 5 steps just mentioned. If you can do that I guarantee you will see success.

Wishing you the best on your journey.

Chad Scott

References

---

[1] 2018 Global Wellness Economy Monitor
https://globalwellnessinstitute.org/industry-research/2018-global-wellness-economy-monitor/

[2] How are habits formed: Modeling habit formation in the real world
Phillipa Lally, Cornelia H. M. van Jarsveld, Henry W. W. Potts, Jane Wardle European Journal of Social Psychology: 16 July 2009
doi.org/10.1002/ejsp.674

[3] Katz DL (2003). "Pandemic obesity and the contagion of nutritional nonsense". *Public Health Rev.* **31** (1): 33–44. PMID 14656042.

[4] Hernández-Alonso P, et al. (2016). High dietary protein intake is associated with an increased body weight and total death risk.
DOI:10.1016/j.clnu.2015.03.016

[5] Gudzune, KA; Doshi, RS; Mehta, AK; Chaudhry, ZW; Jacobs, DK; Vakil, RM; Lee, CJ; Bleich, SN; Clark, JM (7 April 2015). "Efficacy of commercial weight-loss programs: an updated systematic review". *Annals of Internal Medicine.* **162** (7): 501–12. doi: 10.7326/M14-2238. PMC 4446719. PMID 25844997. Atkins resulted in 0.1% to 2.9% greater weight loss at 12 months than counseling.

[6] Alters S, Schiff W (22 February 2012). *Chapter 10: Body Weight and Its Management. Essential Concepts for Healthy Living* (Sixth ed.). Jones & Bartlett Publishers. p. 327. ISBN 978-1-4496-3062-1.

[7] Keith M. Diaz, PhD; Virginia J. Howard, PhD; Brent Hutto, MSPH; Natalie Colabianchi, PhD; John E. Vena, PhD; Monika M. Safford, MD; Steven N. Blair, PED; Steven P. Hooker, PhD. Patterns of Sedentary Behavior and Mortality in U.S. Middle-Aged and Older Adults: A National Cohort Study - Annals of Internal Medicine 3 OCTOBER 2017

[8] Lisa S. Blackwell Columbia University Kali H. Trzesniewski and Carol Sorich Dweck. Implicit theories of intelligence predict achievement across an adolescent transition: a longitudinal study and an intervention. *Child Dev.* 2007 Jan-Feb;78(1):246-63. Stanford University

[9] https://www.ncbi.nlm.nih.gov/pmc/articles/PMC3341916/

[10] Erin Fothergill, Juen Guo, Lilian Howard, Jennifer C. Kerns, Nicolas D. Knuth, Robert Brychta, Kong Y. Chen, Monica C. Skarulis, Mary Walter, Peter J. Walter, Kevin D. Hall. Persistent metabolic adaptation 6 years after "The Biggest Loser" competition. First published: 02 May 2016 doi.org/10.1002/oby.21538

[11]

https://jamanetwork.com/journals/jamainternalmedicine/fullarticle/1392494

[12] https://www.pnas.org/content/109/16/5995

[13] https://n.neurology.org/content/82/16/1395

[14] https://www.ncbi.nlm.nih.gov/pmc/articles/PMC4202343/

[15] Joseph F. Signorile et al, "Difference in muscle activation patterns during high-speed versus standard-speed yoga: A randomized sequence crossover study." Complementary Therapies in Medicine, February 2017, dx.doi.or/10.1016/j.ctim.2016.11.002

[16] Joseph F. Signorile et al, " Differences in Energy Expenditure during high speed versus standard-speed yoga." Complementary Therapies in Medicine, December 2016, DOI: dx.doi.org/10.1016/j.ctim.2016.10.002

[17] https://www.ncbi.nlm.nih.gov/pubmed/17991697

[18] https://www.ncbi.nlm.nih.gov/pubmed/9809557

[19] Effect of Physical Activity on Cognitive Function in Older Adults at Risk for Alzheimer Disease A Randomized Trial
Nicola T. Lautenschlager, MD; Kay L. Cox, PhD; Leon Flicker, MBBS, PhD; et alJonathan K. Foster, DPhil; Frank M. van Bockxmeer, PhD; Jianguo Xiao, MD, PhD; Kathryn R. Greenop, PhD; Osvaldo P. Almeida, MD, PhD
Author Affiliations September 3, 2008 JAMA. 2008;300(9):1027-1037. doi:10.1001/jama.300.9.1027

[20] https://www.unm.edu/~lkravitz/Article folder/musclesgrowLK.html

[21] https://link.springer.com/article/10.1007/BF00423247

[22] https://pubmed.ncbi.nlm.nih.gov/2796409/

[23] Testosterone and the Heart Michael Kirby, Geoffrey Hackett, and Sudarshan Ramachandran Published online 2019 Jul 11. doi: 10.15420/ecr.2019.13.1

[24] https://www.ncbi.nlm.nih.gov/pmc/articles/PMC6765788/

[25] https://www.ncbi.nlm.nih.gov/pmc/articles/PMC5649360/

[26] Resistance Exercise Reverses Aging in Human Skeletal Muscle Simon Melov, Mark A. Tarnopolsky, Kenneth Beckman, Krysta Felkey and Alan Hubbard Published online 2007 May 23. doi: 10.1371/journal.pone.0000465

[27] https://www.ncbi.nlm.nih.gov/pmc/articles/PMC6279907/

[28] Comparisons of Resistance Training and "Cardio" Exercise Modalities as Countermeasures to Microgravity-Induced Physical Deconditioning: New Perspectives and Lessons Learned From Terrestrial Studies James Steele, Patroklos Androulakis-Korakakis, Craig Perrin, James Peter Fisher, Paulo Gentil, Christopher Scott, and André Rosenberger Front Physiol. 2019; 10: 1150. Published online 2019 Sep 10. doi: 10.3389/fphys.2019.01150

[29] https://www.e-jer.org/journal/view.php?number=2013600518

[30] https://www.afcpe.org/news-and-publications/the-standard/2018-3/the-power-of-accountability/

[31] Kraemer W, Fry A, Warren B, et al. Acute Hormonal Responses in Elite Junior Weightlifters. Int J Sports Med. 1992;13(02):103-109. doi:10.1055/s-2007-1021240.

[32] Total Knee Replacement Statistics 2017: Younger Patients Driving Growth iData research 18/07/2018

[33] Bressel E, Willardson JM, Thompson B, Fontana FE. Effect of instruction, surface stability, and load intensity on trunk muscle activity. J Electromyogr Kinesiol. 2009;19(6):e500-e504. doi:10.1016/j.jelekin.2008.10.006.

[34] Schoenfeld BJ, Ratamess NA, Peterson MD, Contreras B, Sonmez GT, Alvar BA. Effects of Different Volume-Equated Resistance Training Loading Strategies on Muscular Adaptations in Well-Trained Men. J Strength Cond Res. 2014;28(10):2909-2918. doi:10.1519/ JSC.0000000000000480.

[35] Schoenfeld BJ, Grgic J, Ogborn D, Krieger JW. Strength and Hypertrophy Adaptations Between Low- vs. High-Load Resistance Training. J Strength Cond Res. 2017;31(12):3508-3523. doi:10.1519/JSC.0000000000002200.

[36] Finn HT, Brennan SL, Gonano BM, et al. Muscle Activation Does Not Increase After a Fatigue Plateau Is Reached During 8 Sets of Resistance Exercise in Trained Individuals. J Strength Cond Res. 2014;28(5):1226-1234. doi:10.1097/JSC.0000000000000226; Hooper DR, Szivak TK, Comstock BA, et al. Effects of Fatigue From Resistance Training on Barbell Back Squat Biomechanics. J Strength Cond Res. 2014;28(4):1127-1134. doi:10.1097/JSC.0000000000000237.

[37] Hatfield DL, Kraemer WJ, Spiering BA, et al. The Impact of Velocity of Movement on Performance Factors in Resistance Exercise. J Strength Cond Res. 2006;20(4):760. doi:10.1519/R-155552.1; Goldberg AL, Etlinger JD, Goldspink DF, Jablecki C. Mechanism of work-induced hypertrophy of skeletal muscle. Med Sci Sports. 1975;7(3):185-198.

[38] Neils CM, Udermann BE, Brice GA, Winchester JB, McGuigan MR. Influence of Contraction Velocity in Untrained Individuals Over the Initial Early Phase of Resistance Training. J Strength Cond Res. 2005;19(4):883. doi:10.1519/R-15794.1.

[39] Munn J, Herbert RD, Hancock MJ, Gandevia SC. Resistance training for strength: effect of number of sets and contraction speed. Med Sci Sports Exerc. 2005;37(9):1622-1626.

[40] Carpinelli RN, Otto RM. Strength training. Single versus multiple sets. Sports Med. 1998;26(2):73-84. doi:10.2165/00007256-199826020-00002

[41] Rhea MR, Alvar BA, Ball SD, Burkett LN. Three sets of weight training superior to 1 set with equal intensity for eliciting strength. J Strength Cond Res. 2002;16(4):525-9.

[42] Krieger JW. Single versus multiple sets of resistance exercise: a meta-regression. J Strength Cond Res. 2009;23(6):1890-901. doi:10.1519/JSC.0b013e3181b370be

[43] Krieger JW. Single vs. multiple sets of resistance exercise for muscle hypertrophy: a meta-analysis. J Strength Cond Res. 2010;24(4):1150-9. doi:10.1519/JSC.0b013e3181d4d436

[44] Souza-Junior TP, Willardson JM, Bloomer R, et al. Strength and hypertrophy responses to constant and decreasing rest intervals in trained men using creatine supplementation. J Int Soc Sports Nutr. 2011;8(1):17. doi:10.1186/1550-2783-8-17.

[45] Radaelli R, Fleck SJ, Leite T, et al. Dose-Response of 1, 3, and 5 Sets of Resistance Exercise on Strength, Local Muscular Endurance, and Hypertrophy. J Strength Cond Res. 2015;29(5):1349-1358. doi:10.1519/JSC.0000000000000758;

Robbins DW, Marshall PW, McEwen M. The Effect of Training Volume on Lower-Body Strength. J Strength Cond Res. 2012;26(1):34-39. doi:10.1519/ JSC.0b013e31821d5cc4.

[46] De Salles BF, Simão R, Miranda F, da Silva Novaes J, Lemos A, Willardson JM. Rest Interval between Sets in Strength Training. Sport Med. 2009;39(9):765-777. doi:10.2165/11315230-000000000-00000.

[47] Willardson JM, Burkett LN. The Effect of Different Rest Intervals Between Sets on Volume Components and Strength Gains. J Strength Cond Res. 2008;22(1):146-152. doi:10.1519/JSC.0b013e31815f912d.

[48] Kujala UM, Kvist M, Osterman K. Knee injuries in athletes. Review of exertion injuries and retrospective study of outpatient sports clinic material. Sports Med. 3(6):447-460; Maffulli N, Longo UG, Gougoulias N, Caine D, Denaro V. Sport injuries: a review of outcomes. Br Med Bull. 2011;97(1):47-80. doi:10.1093/bmb/ldq026.

[49] Robbins DW, Marshall PW, McEwen M. The Effect of Training Volume on Lower-Body Strength. J Strength Cond Res. 2012;26(1):34-39. doi:10.1519/JSC.0b013e31821d5cc4.

[50] https://www.sciencedirect.com/science/article/abs/pii/S030698770700566X

[51] http://onlinelibrary.wiley.com/doi/10.1002/14651858.CD008262.pub2/abstract

[52] https://www.sciencedirect.com/science/article/abs/pii/0891584994900302

[53] https://www.ncbi.nlm.nih.gov/pmc/articles/PMC5025014/

[54] Kreher JB, Schwartz JB. Overtraining syndrome: a practical guide. Sports Health. 2012;4(2):128-138. doi:10.1177/1941738111434406.

[55] Kreher JB. Diagnosis and prevention of overtraining syndrome: an opinion on education strategies. Open access J Sport Med. 2016;7:115-122. doi:10.2147/OAJSM.S91657.

[56] Fradkin AJ, Zazryn TR, Smoliga JM. Effects of warming-up on physical performance: a systematic review with meta-analysis. J strength Cond Res. 2010;24(1):140-148. doi:10.1519/JSC.0b013e3181c643a0.

[57] G Kirkwood, H Rampes, V Tuffrey, J Richardson, K Pilkington, and S Ramaratnam Yoga for anxiety: a systematic review of the

research evidence Br J Sports Med. 2005 Dec; 39(12): 884–891. doi: 10.1136/bjsm.2005.018069

[58] G. L. Moseley and D.S. Butler, "Fifteen Years of Explaining Pain: The Past, Present, and Future," Jpain 16(2015)
[59] M.C. Bushnell et al, "Cognitive and emotional control of pain and its disruption in chronic pain," Nat Rev Neurosci 14(2015)

[60] Sherman, G. D., Lerner, J. S., Josephs, R. A., Renshon, J., & Gross, J. J. (2016). The interaction of testosterone and cortisol is associated with attained status in male executives. *Journal of Personality and Social Psychology, 110*(6), 921-929. doi.10.1037/pspp0000063

[61] Assessment of stresses in the cervical spine caused by posture and position of the head, K. K. Hansraj, *Surg Tech Int* 25 (2014)

[62] A pragmatic Multicentered Randomized Controlled Trial of Yoga for Chronic Low Back Pain; Economic Evaluation, L-H Chuang et al, *Spine* 37 (2012)

[63] A simple questionnaire to detect hyper mobility: an adjunct to the assessment of patients with diffuse musculoskeletal pain," Intl J Clin Pract 57 (2003); G.N. Kawchuk et all

[64] "Real-Time Visualsation of Joint Cavitation, " PLoS ONE 10(2015); V.K. Ranganathan et al

[65] Is high-intensity interval training a time-efficient exercise strategy to improve health and fitness? Gillen JB1, Gibala MJ. Appli Physial Ntur Metab 2014 Mar;39(3):409-12. doi: 10.1139/apnm-2013-0187. Epub 2013 Sep 27.

[66] http://www.ncbi.nlm.nih.gov/pubmed/22946099

[67] The exercise-induced growth hormone response in athletes. Godfrey RJ, Madowick Z, Whyte GP. Sports Med. 2003;33(8):599-613.

[68] The time course of the human growth hormone response to a 6 s and a 30 s cycle ergometer sprint. Stokes KA, Nevill ME, Hall GM, Lakomv HK J Sports Sci. 2002 Jun;20(6):487-94.

[69] https://www.ncbi.nlm.nih.gov/pmc/articles/PMC2992225/

[70] https://www.ncbi.nlm.nih.gov/pubmed/27172268

[71] https://www.ncbi.nlm.nih.gov/pmc/articles/PMC3463487/

72
https://www.sciencedirect.com/science/article/abs/pii/S00319384140
05095

73 Biolo G, Tipton KD, Klein S, Wolfe RR. An abundant supply of amino acids enhances the metabolic effect of exercise on muscle protein. Am J Physiol Metab. 1997;273(1):E122-E129. doi:10.1152/ajpendo.1997.273.1.E122. Matthews, Michael. Bigger Leaner Stronger: The Simple Science of Building the Ultimate Male Body (Muscle for Life Book 1) (p. 194). Oculus Publishers. Kindle Edition.
74 Jeukendrup AE, Killer SC. The Myths Surrounding Pre-Exercise Carbohydrate Feeding. Ann Nutr Metab. 2010;57(s2):18-25. doi:10.1159/000322698; Hargreaves M, Hawley JA, Jeukendrup A. Pre-exercise carbohydrate and fat ingestion: effects on metabolism and performance. J Sports Sci. 2004;22(1):31-38. doi:10.1080/0264041031000140536.

75 http://jap.physiology.org/content/106/6/2026.short

76 https://jissn.biomedcentral.com/articles/10.1186/1550-2783-10-5

77 http://europepmc.org/article/med/12750588

78 https://www.ncbi.nlm.nih.gov/pmc/articles/PMC5384055/

79 https://www.ncbi.nlm.nih.gov/pmc/articles/PMC524355/

80 Schoenfeld BJ, Ratamess NA, Peterson MD, Contreras B, Sonmez GT, Alvar BA. Effects of Different Volume-Equated Resistance Training Loading Strategies on Muscular Adaptations in Well- Trained Men. J Strength Cond Res. 2014;28(10):2909-2918. doi:10.1519/JSC.0000000000000480.

81 Biolo G, Tipton KD, Klein S, Wolfe RR. An abundant supply of amino acids enhances the metabolic effect of exercise on muscle protein. Am J Physiol Metab. 1997;273(1):E122-E129. doi:10.1152/ajpendo.1997.273.1.E122. Matthews, Michael. Bigger Leaner Stronger: The Simple Science of Building the Ultimate Male Body (Muscle for Life Book 1) (p. 194). Oculus Publishers. Kindle Edition.

82 https://www.ncbi.nlm.nih.gov/pmc/articles/PMC4989512/

83 https://www.ncbi.nlm.nih.gov/pmc/articles/PMC2905334/

84 https://www.afcpe.org/news-and-publications/the-standard/2018-3/the-power-of-accountability/